home herbal
remedies

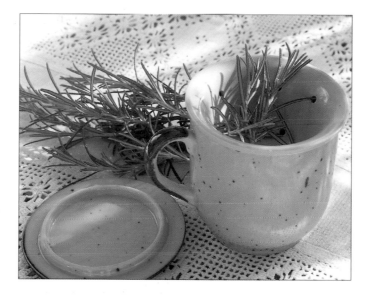

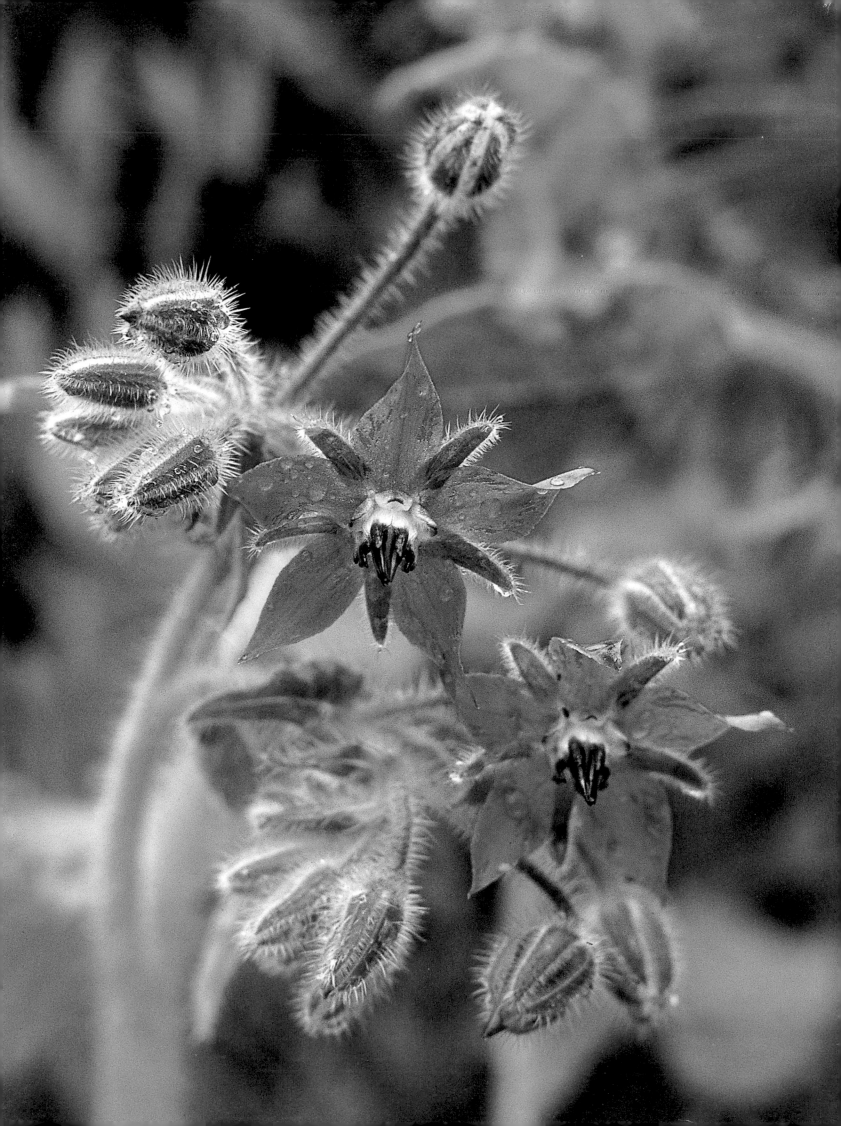

home herbal remedies

Making natural preparations for boosting health and treating common ailments, with over 300 photographs

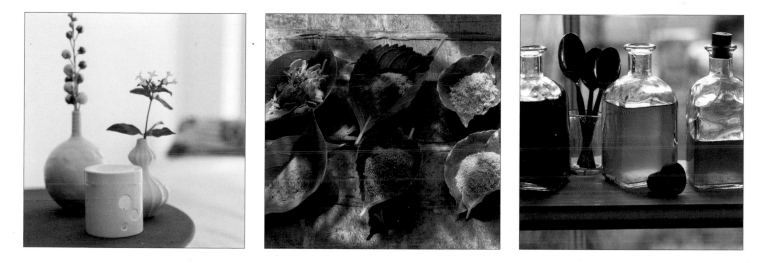

JESSICA HOUDRET

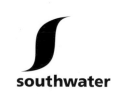

southwater

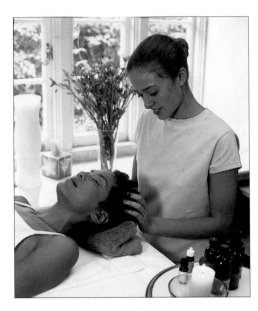
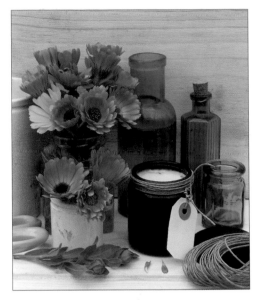
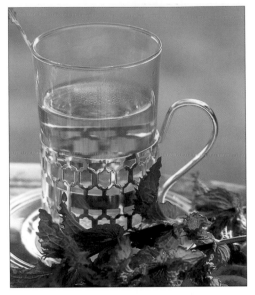

This edition is published by Southwater, an imprint of Anness Publishing Ltd, Blaby Road, Wigston, Leicestershire LE18 4SE

info@anness.com;
www.southwaterbooks.com;
www.annesspublishing.com

If you like the images in this book and would like to investigate using them for publishing, promotions or advertising, please visit our website www.practicalpictures.com for more information.

Publisher: Joanna Lorenz
Editorial director: Helen Sudell
Editor: Simona Hill
Designer: Nigel Partridge
Production controller: Christine Ni

ETHICAL TRADING POLICY
Because of our ongoing ecological investment programme, you, as our customer, have the reassurance of knowing that a tree is being cultivated to naturally replace the materials used to make this book. For further information about this scheme, go to www.annesspublishing.com/trees

The directory of herbs was previously published as part of a larger volume, *The Illustrated Guide to Herbal Home Remedies*

DISCLAIMER
This book is intended as a source of information on herbs and their uses, and does not provide recommendations as a replacement for professional medical advice and treatment. The publishers and the author cannot accept responsibility for any specific individual's reactions, nor for any harmful or ill effects or damage, arising from the use of the general data and suggestions here, whether in remedy form or otherwise. Nor is any responsibility taken for mistaken identity or inappropriate use of the plants. It is always advisable to consult a medical practitioner or qualified medical herbalist before using herbal treatments or remedies, particularly if you are pregnant, suffering from an ongoing medical condition or taking any other medication.

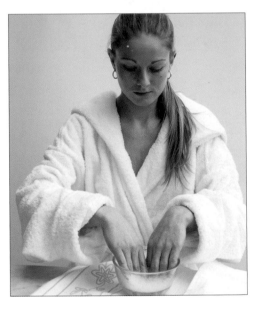
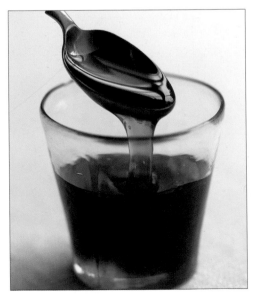

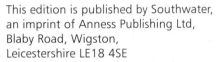

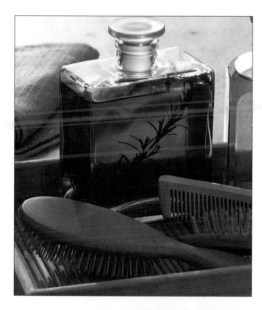

CONTENTS

Introduction 6

USING MEDICINAL HERBS 8
How Safe are Herbal
  Remedies? 10
Quality Control and Dosage 12
Wild Herbs 14
Garden Herbs 15
Growing Herbs in the Garden 16
Harvesting, Drying and Storing 18
Other Herbal Remedy
  Ingredients 20
Essential Oils 22
Aromatherapy 24
Making Infusions 26
Making Decoctions
  and Syrups 27
Making Tinctures 28
Making Cold-infused Oils 29
Making Poultices
  and Compresses 30
Making Creams
  and Ointments 31
Making Inhalations 32
Making Bath Mixes and
  Sleep Pillows 33
Healing Herbs in Food 34

**HERBAL REMEDIES FOR
COMMON AILMENTS 36**
Anxiety 38
Stress 39
Depression and
  Feeling Low 40
Poor Memory and
  Concentration 41
Tiredness and Low Energy 42
Sleep Disturbances 43
Headaches 44
Migraine 45
Colds and Influenza 46
Coughs 48
Sore Throats 49

Catarrh 50
Hayfever 51
Indigestion 52
Acidity and Heartburn 53
Nausea and Vomiting 54
Mouth Ulcers 55
Constipation 56
Diarrhoea 57
Poor Circulation 58
Cold Hands and Feet 59
Chilblains 60
Cramp 61
Skin Irritations 62
Eczema 63
Acne 64
Athlete's Foot 65
Boils and Abscesses 66
Cold Sores 67
Eye Strain 68
Styes 69
Menstrual Problems 70
Pre-menstrual Symptoms 71
Menopausal Problems 72
Rheumatism and Arthritis 74
Bites and Stings 76
Cuts and Grazes 77
Bruises 78
Sprains and Strains 79
Burns 80
Sunburn 81

**HERBAL BEAUTY
TREATMENTS 82**
Healthy Hair 84
Facial Care 86
Eyes and Lips 88
Teeth and Fresh Breath 89
Hands and Nails 90
Foot Treatments 91
Skin Treatments 92
Bathing 94

Index 96

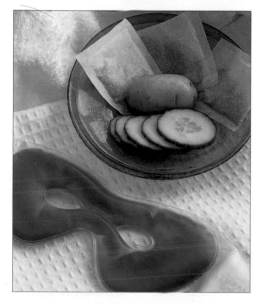

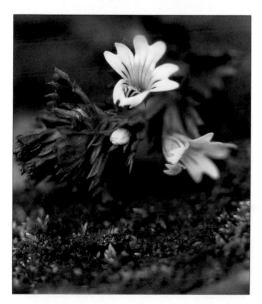

Introduction

Herbs and home remedies can play a major role in promoting health and well-being. They are often effective in alleviating the symptoms of everyday illnesses, such as coughs and colds or aches and pains, and are useful as first aid for a range of minor accidents, from cuts and grazes to insect bites and stings.

This book is intended as a practical guide to using herbs in the home as part of a healthy way of living. In order to do so to best advantage, it helps to understand how herbal remedies work and why.

Self-treatment is sensible and appropriate for everyday ailments, or for relieving the discomfort of ongoing conditions that are not critical. However, for more serious problems it should never take the place of professional medical advice. If you stub your toe, a comfrey poultice is a good way to take away the pain, but if you develop bronchitis or pneumonia, you must consult your doctor.

Herbal medicine may also be appropriate where a specific condition is not responding to orthodox medical treatment. But in such a case self-treatment is again unwise, and you should consult a qualified herbal practitioner for proper advice on which herbal treatments would be best for your individual requirements.

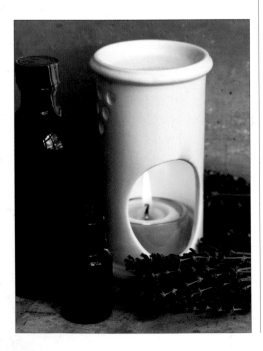

How herbal remedies work

Plants have been used as medicine for centuries, and modern research has confirmed the therapeutic properties of many. Some contain potent alkaloids and other constituents, which is why they work effectively and why many of them form the basis of modern pharmaceutical drugs. It is also why some of them may interact with pharmaceutical drugs. But there is a difference between using the most powerful constituent of a herb, isolated and extracted in a laboratory and usually synthesized (as in pharmaceutical drugs), and using a home preparation made from the whole plant. Herbs should always be used with care in home remedies, and warnings respected.

The constituents of herbs cause them to act on the body in a variety of ways. Some have a sedative action; others are stimulants. There are those that enhance the circulation of blood, and those with an astringent action, which means that they constrict bodily tissues and are useful in healing cuts and wounds. Some herbs have a detoxifying effect, helping to eliminate toxins and waste from the system, and some stimulate digestion and aid the absorption of nutrients. Many more fight infections, due to their antiseptic, antibacterial or antifungal properties, and a few have more complex actions, such as regulating hormonal activity.

Herbal remedies remain a valuable resource for many minor ills, but it would be foolish to ignore scientific advances and not to take advantage of modern medical knowledge when dealing with more serious health conditions.

Herbs for general well-being

No alternative therapy should be seen as a quick cure-all to be taken in isolation. For herbal remedies to have any impact they must be part of a healthy lifestyle. It's a question of "rounding up all the usual suspects": paying attention to diet, not

Left *Essential oils, such as lavender, can be used in aromatherapy to lift the mood and aid relaxation.*

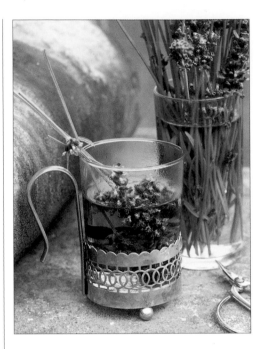

Above *Infusions are a simple way to enjoy the benefits of herbs.*

smoking, not drinking too much, taking exercise and regulating stress by finding time for relaxation techniques.

This is where herbs also play an important role. They are vital as agents for maintaining general well-being. Incorporating them in food adds flavour and interest, making it easier to keep to a healthy diet, as well as providing an opportunity to benefit from their intrinsic properties. In beauty products they provide the ingredients for a range of simple preparations to make at home, which may be used to supplement or replace commercially manufactured beauty products, many of which can contain potentially harmful chemicals. These may be present in only small amounts in each individual product, but the effect can be cumulative, and changing to a herbal beauty regime is all part of a healthy lifestyle based on holistic principles.

Right *Dried leafy herbs and flowers have plenty of uses around the home as well as having a therapeutic use in many herbal remedies. Growing herbs, harvesting, drying and then using them is rewarding and can be life-enhancing.*

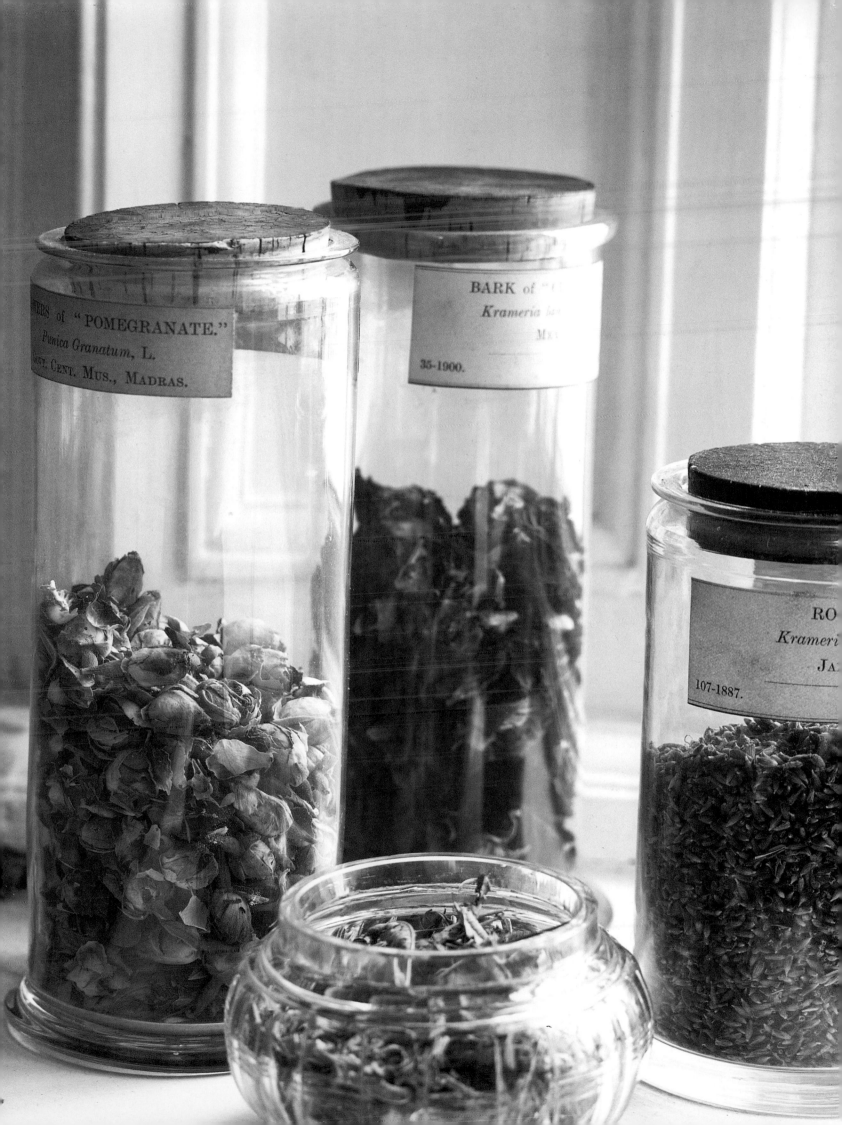

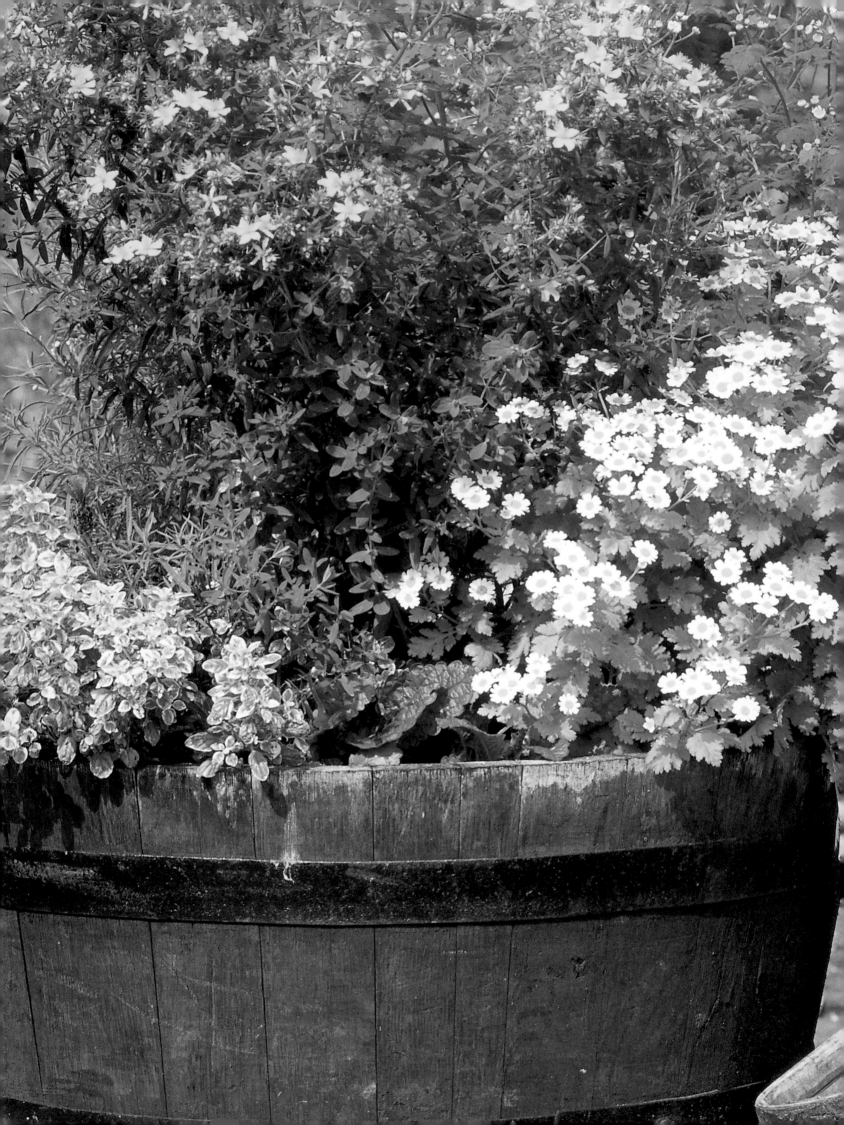

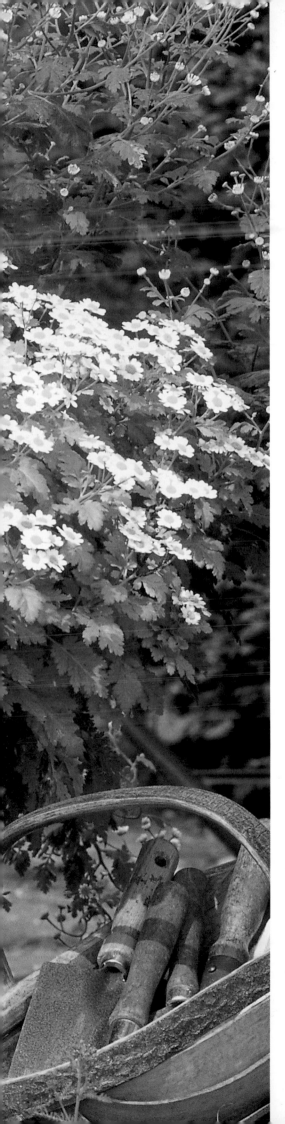

Using Medicinal Herbs

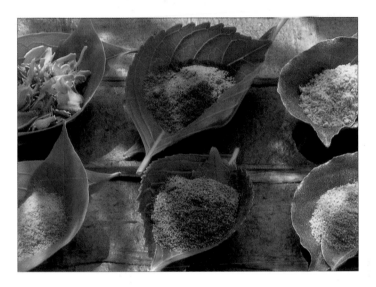

Medicinal herbs have been used throughout history to cure ills and promote well-being. Despite huge advances in modern medical science, they remain popular today, with 80 per cent of the world's population relying on herbal medicine for primary healthcare. Safety is an important issue, however, and it should be stressed that these plants are effective because they contain potent constituents. Dosages, diagnosis and quality of product are crucial and it is vital to remember that herbs can interact with pharmaceutical drugs. If in doubt as to what to take and when, professional guidance should be sought. Used sensibly and with care, medicinal herbs can greatly add to the quality of life.

Above *Many herbs and spices have antibacterial properties.*

Left *Growing herbs can be an attractive talking point in the garden, as well as providing fresh material for your medicinal requirements.*

How Safe are Herbal Remedies?

There is a lot of controversy over the safety of herbal remedies, with new research constantly highlighting potential risks and previously unsuspected side effects. It is as well to remember that this also applies to medical drugs, food and drink, and many of the products we use in our everyday lives. Reports appear, almost daily, on newly discovered health risks in these areas.

The truth is that if taken with due care and in the correct dosage, herbal remedies have a good safety record. Self-diagnosis and self-treatment can be hazardous however, and there are a number of factors to take into account before taking any herbal remedies. None of the remedies suggested in this book are intended to replace professional medical treatment or advice, and it is always best to speak to your doctor before embarking on any alternative therapy.

Toxic plants

Just because something is "natural" does not mean it is good for you. Some natural substances, including plants, are highly toxic

Below Before you use any medicinal plant you have gathered yourself, make sure that you have identified it correctly.

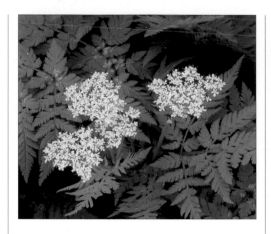

Above *The leaves of sweet cicely (*Myrrhis odorata*) are edible.*

to humans. Correct identification is crucial when picking herbs to use in herbal preparations. Some toxic plants resemble others that are harmless. For example, cow parsley and hemlock, which are poisonous, bear a strong resemblance to sweet cicely (*Myrrhis odorata*), a delightful herb that can be used to add sweetness to food.

Side effects

Some herbs may cause side effects, such as gastro-intestinal upsets, headaches or rashes. A few may have more serious adverse effects, including liver damage, usually in

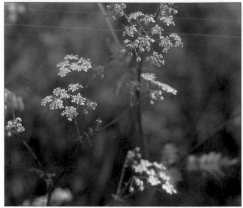

Above *Cow parsley (*Anthriscus sylvestris*) should not be confused with sweet cicely.*

rare cases or when taken in large amounts. At the first sign of any adverse reaction, stop taking the herb immediately and consult a qualified herbalist or medical practitioner.

Others, including seemingly innocuous plants such as pot marigold (*Calendula officinalis*), may cause allergic reactions in certain people. For anyone prone to allergies, it is sensible to start with a small amount of any herbal product, and then step up the dose if all seems well.

Below Drinking plenty of water is essential for good health.

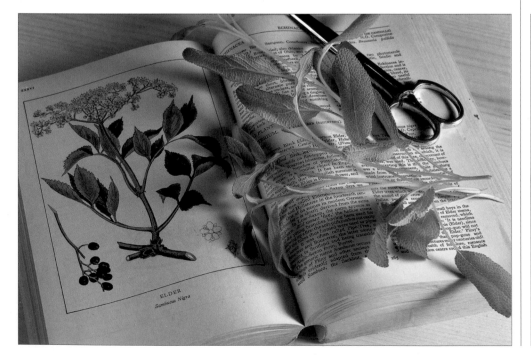

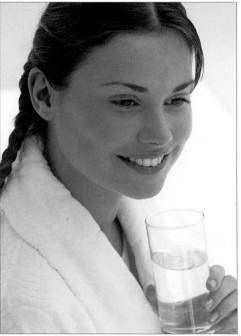

Contra-indications

Some illnesses and pre-existing health conditions can be made worse by a specific herb, so if herbs are to be taken medicinally, try each first to ensure there are no adverse reactions. Liquorice (*Glycyrrhiza glabra*), for example, can increase high blood pressure through its action on the adrenal glands. As some people may be unaware that their blood pressure is raised when they are taking a remedy for a different condition, it is generally unwise to use liquorice in herbal preparations. For this reason it does not feature in any recipes in this book, despite its otherwise beneficial properties.

Safety checklist

- Remember that "natural" does not necessarily mean "safe".
- Check that you have correctly identified herbs for use in remedies.
- Buy dried herbs and herbal products from a reliable source.
- Do not exceed recommended doses.
- Remember that some herbs are safe in low doses but toxic in large doses.
- Do not take any herbal remedy continuously for more than 2–3 weeks.
- Do not use poultices or compresses continuously for more than 1–2 days.
- If prone to allergies, start by taking a low dose, gradually increasing it if no adverse reaction is experienced.
- Do not take essential oils internally.
- If you experience any adverse reaction to a herbal remedy, seek professional advice immediately.
- Herbal remedies should not be taken if elderly, or pregnant, or by young children without professional advice.
- If you have a pre-existing health condition, including high blood pressure, seek medical advice before taking herbal remedies.
- If you are taking pharmaceutical drugs or prescribed medication, seek medical advice before taking herbal remedies.

CAUTION Pharmaceutical drugs include many common over-the-counter products, such as aspirin, as well as prescribed medicines.

So many herbs are contra-indicated during pregnancy or when breastfeeding that it is wisest not to take any at such times, especially in larger, medicinal doses, without first seeking professional advice.

Interactions

Some herbs may interact with certain pharmaceutical drugs, usually by increasing or decreasing their effect, although this is rare in practice. Some interactions may be minor, but others can be life-threatening. St John's wort (*Hypericum perforatum*), hailed until fairly recently as the natural way to treat depression without the side effects of many medical antidepressant drugs, has since been found to interact with vital medically prescribed drugs for other conditions, and can therefore no longer be recommended for internal use in home remedies or for self-treatment.

Herbal remedies and pharmaceutical drugs are not necessarily mutually exclusive, but decisions on taking both at the same time should be left to professionals. The rule is simple: never take herbal remedies at the same time as prescribed medication without telling your doctor. Equally, a professional herbal consultant should always be informed during a consultation of any pharmaceutical drugs you are taking. The main categories of pharmaceutical drugs that may be affected by herbal preparations are: anticoagulants (blood-thinning drugs, including aspirin and warfarin); antidepressants; drugs for epilepsy; medication for diabetes; drugs used to treat heart disorders; immuno-suppressants; the contraceptive pill; HRT and fertility treatment.

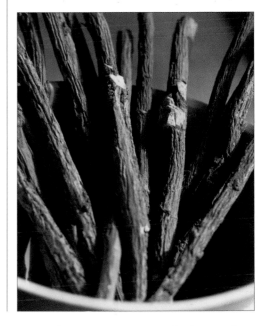

Below *Liquorice may raise blood pressure if taken in large, medicinal doses.*

Herb–drug interactions

This list includes some herbs commonly used as remedies, and the main categories of pharmaceutical medicines with which they may interact:

Herb	Drugs that may be affected
• Angelica (*Angelica archangelica*)	anticoagulants
• Chaste tree (*Vitex agnus-castus*)	contraceptive pill, fertility treatment, HRT
• Devil's claw (*Harpagophytum procumbens*)	various
• Echinacea (*Echinacea angustifolia, E. purpurea*)	various
• Evening primrose (*Oenothera biennis*)	epilepsy drugs
• Feverfew (*Tanacetum parthenium*)	anticoagulants
• Fenugreek (*Trigonella foenum-graecum*)	anticoagulants, diabetic medicine
• Garlic (*Allium sativum*)	anticoagulants
• Ginger (*Zingiber officinalis*)	anticoagulants
• Ginseng (*Panax ginseng*)	high blood pressure, diabetes medication
• Hawthorn (*Crataegus* spp)	high blood pressure, heart medication
• St John's wort (*Hypericum perforatum*)	contraceptive pill, immuno-suppressants
• Turmeric (*Curcuma longa*)	anticoagulants
• Valerian (*Valeriana officinalis*)	epilepsy drugs

Quality Control and Dosage

Using herbs safely is not just about finding the correct remedy. It's vital to be confident about the quality of the ingredients and to observe the guidelines on dosage.

Home-grown herbs and remedies

There are many advantages to using herbs you have grown yourself, not least that you will know the plant material is clean, and has not been mixed with soil or other species or sprayed with pesticides. If you dry your own herbs, you will know how old they are and that they have not been adulterated with suspect material. All these things can be enormously reassuring.

Buying herbs for use in remedies

Quality is more of an issue when it comes to buying dried herbs to make your own preparations. Herb crops are subject to natural variation, due to changing weather and growing conditions, and some batches will be of higher quality than others. More seriously, one of the problems of buying dried herbs is that they are easy to adulterate, and there have been instances when toxic plant material has been accidentally mixed in with beneficial herbs.

Always buy from a reputable source, preferably one where products have been standardized or there is some guarantee of quality control. Remember that this will not apply to all internet sources.

Chinese herbs

There have been some reports of batches of imported Chinese herbs being severely contaminated. At the time of writing there is no reliable way of being sure of their safety, and quality issues on this score remain a health concern.

Below *Growing your own herbs for use in home remedies ensures a safe supply.*

Legislation on herbal products

In the USA, herbal remedies are mostly classified as food supplements and come under regulations for retailing food, rather than medicines. In the European Union and Australia, legislation on quality standards and labelling requirements for herbal medicinal products has been put in place. In Europe, the Traditional Herbal Medicinal Products Directive now requires anything sold as a herbal remedy to be licensed, an extremely costly procedure that will inevitably result in fewer products being available. At present only the components of the remedy may be stated on the label, but by 2011, provided the product is licensed, the manufacturer will be allowed to include information on the ill-health condition it is intended to treat. The legislation is applied to dried herbs only if they are sold as medicines, and of course it does not prevent you growing and using your own herbs.

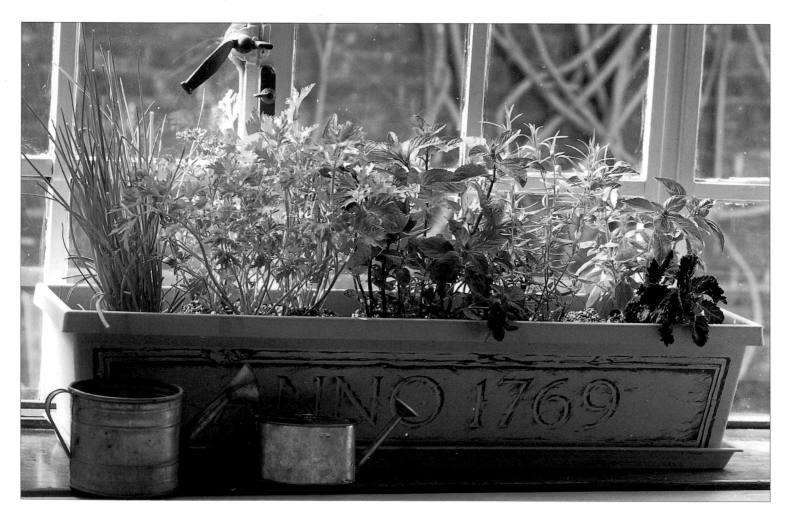

Right *You can dry home-grown herbs to make your own herbal preparations. Choose a warm morning to harvest them, before the essential oils have evaporated.*

Changes and updates are ongoing, and the Medicine Control Agency (dedicated to safety issues associated with herbal medicines) reviews the current situation on its website.

Sensible dosages

Anything, including water and carrot juice, can be harmful if taken in vast quantities. How much you take of any herb, and in what form or concentration, is crucial to safety. Taking more of a herbal product to remedy a particular problem, far from making it better more quickly, is likely to make things worse. Some herbs, even culinary herbs such as sage, are perfectly safe in normal, recommended quantities, but toxic in large amounts. Herbal preparations work gently on the system, and results may not be felt immediately. It is important that herbs should be taken only in the quantities recommended and, for maximum effect, in conjunction with a healthy lifestyle. Doses need to be carefully monitored when taking herbs as extracts or in manufactured medicinal preparations, and essential oils should not be taken internally without professional advice. (See the guidelines for standard adult doses.) Always follow guidelines carefully and use common sense when taking herbal remedies. It is no good expecting herbal remedies to work if you take no exercise and eat badly.

Below *Consult a healthcare professional for advice before taking herbal remedies.*

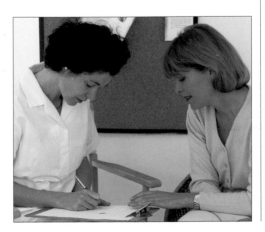

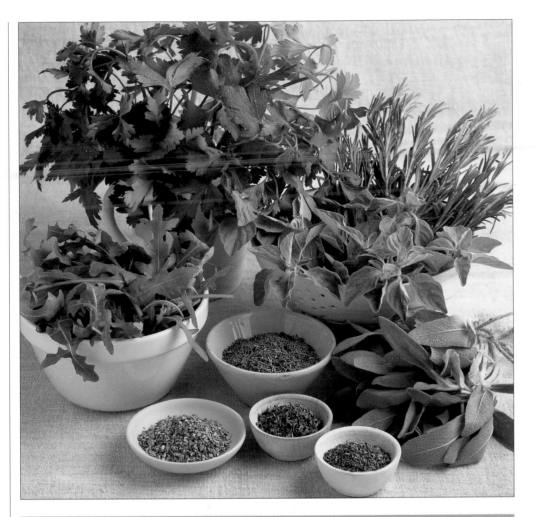

Guidelines for standard adult doses

For children under 12 and the elderly, seek the advice of a professional herbalist before using herbal remedies.

• Infusions (teas): 1 cup 3 times daily.
• Decoctions: 1 cup 3 times daily.
• Syrups: 5–10ml/1 2 tsp 3 times daily.
• Tinctures (home-made): 5ml/1 tsp diluted in a little water or fruit juice, 3 times daily.
• Tinctures (bought): These vary in strength, and should be taken according to the manufacturer's directions, or following professional advice.
• Capsules (bought): According to manufacturer's directions.
• Compresses: Apply as often as required, for 10–15 minutes at a time (for no longer than 1–2 days).
• Poultices: Apply 2–3 times a day for 2–3 hours at a time (for no longer than 1–2 days).
• Steam inhalations: 2–3 times a day, for up to 10 minutes at a time.
• Essential oils in bath: 5–6 drops.
• Essential oils for massage: 1–2 drops essential oil in 5ml/1 tsp base oil (10–12 drops in 30ml/2 tbsp).
• Essential oils in a vaporizer: 5–8 drops initially, topping up as necessary.

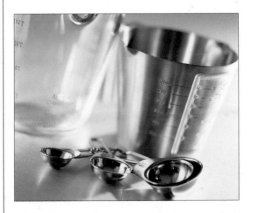

Left *Measuring jugs (cups) and spoons are essential for accurately measuring any remedies that are taken orally. Taking too much may be harmful.*

Wild Herbs

Many medicinal herbs are wild plants, and if you are tempted to pick them for use in home preparations you should be careful to follow the code of conduct for harvesting plants from the wild. Remember that some species are protected by law.

Commercial wild harvesting

Plants for use in commercial herbal medicines and products are still gathered from the wild in parts of Europe and in the developing world. This practice has brought many species to the point of extinction, such as golden seal (*Hydrastis canadensis*) and *Echinacea* in North America. To counteract this trend, some countries have instituted large-scale cultivation of medicinal herb crops, such as German chamomile (*Matricaria recutita*) and *Ginkgo biloba*.

Other useful herbs are familiar as common 'weeds' and as such can be encouraged to grow in the untended areas of your garden, or even cultivated.

Wild herbs to harvest

• **Chickweed** (*Stellaria media*) – A creeping ground-cover plant, rich in vitamins, which comes up in cleared ground in spring.
• **Cleavers** (*Galium aparine*) – It is tempting to pull out this prolific, sticky creeper as

Below *Dandelions have many uses in herbal remedies.*

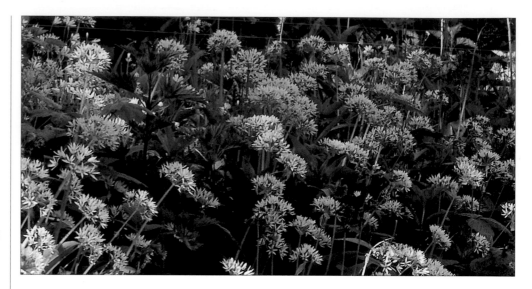

Above *Herbs with medicinal properties can be found growing wild in many different plant habitats.*

soon as you see it, but leave a patch to grow over a wall or fence for use as a spring tonic.
• **Dandelion** (*Taraxacum officinale*) – An easy plant to cultivate, its cheery yellow flowers feature in spring and summer. It self-seeds freely and even if the whole plant is dug up it will regenerate from a tiny portion of root left in the soil. The leaves are packed with vitamins and minerals.
• **Stinging nettles** (*Urtica dioica*) – For maximum medicinal potency these should not be grown in rich soil. Allow clumps to flourish where they come up, in a wild corner of the garden.

Below *Elderflowers can be made into soothing teas and lotions.*

• **Yarrow** (*Achillea millefolium*) – A common grassland weed with astringent properties, traditionally used to staunch bleeding, it will be improved if you dig it up and re-plant in cultivated soil. There are many ornamental *Achillea* varieties but they do not have the same medicinal properties as the species.
• **Elder** (*Sambucus nigra*) – If you do not have room in the garden for an elder tree ("the poor man's medicine chest"), this is one that can be harvested from the wild, provided the wild harvesting code of conduct is followed.

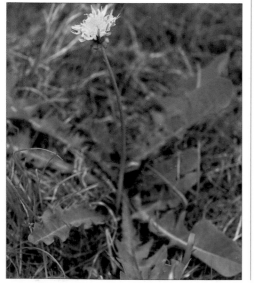

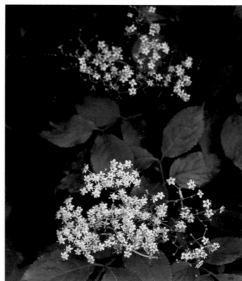

Code of conduct for harvesting from the wild

• Always be sure you have identified the plant correctly.
• Do not pick near roadsides, or at field edges where crops may have been sprayed with pesticides.
• Make sure the plant you pick is not legally protected.
• Never uproot a wild plant.
• Do not always pick from the same area, or where the species is scarce.
• Avoid plants that are stunted or do not look healthy.

Garden Herbs

There are many advantages to growing your own plants for use in herbal preparations:

- You can be sure that they have not been contaminated or sprayed with pesticides.
- Identification is secure (provided you have grown the right variety and labelled it correctly).
- You will have fresh material to hand just when you need it.
- If you are using dried material from herbs you have grown, you can ensure it has not been kept too long.
- You can pick material for drying at the optimum time of day.
- There is a wide range of seeds and plants from which to choose.

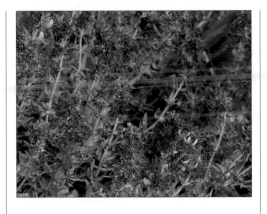

Above *Hyssop* (Hyssopus officinalis*) has colourful flowers and is easy to grow in the garden for use in home remedies. It needs a sunny spot in well-drained soil.*

Herbs to grow in the garden

Plants that can be used in herbal home preparations come from all over the world. Some flourish in tropical climates, but there are a large number that originate from temperate regions and can withstand frost. Tender plants, such as *Aloe vera*, can be successfully grown as houseplants.

The lists below are not exhaustive but will form the basis of a useful collection as the source of fresh ingredients for home-made herbal preparations.

Remember that many herbs fulfil more than one purpose and cannot necessarily be categorized as exclusively medicinal or culinary.

Annuals and biennials

These are best grown from seed.

- Angelica (*Angelica archangelica*)
- Basil (*Ocimum basilicum*)
- Borage (*Borago officinalis*)
- Calendula (*Calendula officinalis*)
- Chervil (*Anthriscus cerefolium*)
- Coriander (*Coriandrum sativum*)
- Wild (German) chamomile (*Matricaria recutita*)
- Parsley (*Petroselinum crispum*)
- Garlic (*Allium sativum*) – grow from a "clove" or small bulblet.

Below *Buy seed from a reputable supplier to be sure of good quality.*

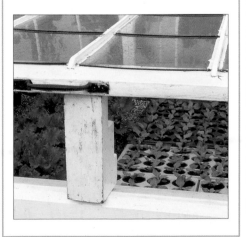

Perennials

It is easier to buy most of these as little plants, or to obtain them as root divisions or offsets from existing plants. Some may also be grown successfully from seed.

- Anise hyssop (*Agastache foeniculum*)
- Boneset (*Eupatorium perfoliatum*)
- Chamomile (*Chamaemelum nobile*)
- Comfrey (*Symphytum officinalis*)
- Cotton lavender (*Santolina chamaecyparissus*)
- Echinacea (*Echinacea purpurea*)
- Elecampane (*Inula helenium*)
- Fennel (*Foeniculum vulgare*)
- Feverfew (*Tanacetum parthenium*)
- Globe artichoke (*Cynara scolymus*)
- Houseleek (*Sempervivum tectorum*)
- Hyssop (*Hyssopus officinalis*)
- St John's wort (*Hypericum perforatum*)
- Lavender (*Lavandula* spp)
- Lemon balm (*Melissa officinalis*)
- Lemon verbena (*Aloysia triphylla*)
- Marjoram (*Origanum* spp)
- Marshmallow (*Althaea officinalis*)
- Mint (*Mentha* spp)
- Rose (*Rosa* spp)
- Rosemary (*Rosmarinus officinalis*)
- Sage (*Salvia officinalis*)
- Soapwort (*Saponaria officinalis*)

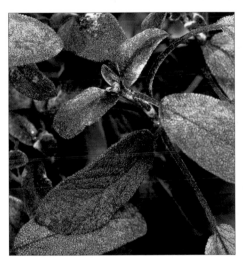

Above *Purple sage* (Salvia officinalis purpurea*) is an attractive sub-shrub.*

- Southernwood (*Artemisia abrotanum*)
- Thyme (*Thymus* spp)
- Valerian (*Valeriana officinalis*)

Climbers
- Hops (*Humulus lupulus*)
- Passion flower (*Passiflora incarnata*)

Shrubs
- Elder (*Sambucus nigra*)
- Witch hazel (*Hamamelis virginiana*)

Growing Herbs in the Garden

A carefully designed and stocked herb garden will provide all the fresh plant material you need for making your own herbal preparations. Herbs are not fussy or difficult plants to grow, but giving them the right soil and situation will ensure that you get the best from them.

Site and soil

A sunny sheltered position and light, dryish soil suits most herbs best. For many of them, the sunnier and hotter the site is, the more fragrance and flavour they will have and the higher will be the proportion of active constituents. The smell and taste of herbs is largely due to the production of essential oils within the plants. If they are grown in hot conditions, the concentrations of essential oils will be greater. Dull, damp conditions and a very moist rich soil will produce lush, leafy plants with a milder flavour and little scent. To cater for moisture lovers, such as angelica (*Angelica archangelica*), add extra organic matter in the area where they grow.

Layout and design

Although herbs can be grown throughout the garden, it is more convenient when using them as ingredients for preparations to plant them together in a designated herb garden. A formal, symmetrical design of small rectangular beds, divided by gravel or paved paths, is a traditional layout that makes tending and harvesting easy. Some beds could be devoted to a single species, in the style of a medieval apothecary's garden, or collections of principally medicinal, culinary or fragrant herbs could be grouped together in larger beds. An informal cottage-garden style provides plenty of scope for imaginative planting and requires a little less maintenance than the more formal designs.

Watering and maintenance

Most herbs will withstand dry summers, but some, such as parsley (*Petroselinum crispum*) and chervil (*Anthriscus cerefolium*), are apt to bolt in dry conditions and may need watering. Herbs with a root system of vigorous runners, such as mint (*Mentha* spp),

can become invasive unless you restrict the roots by growing them in a bucket with the bottom removed, sunk in the soil. Remove heads of rampant seeders, such as lemon balm (*Melissa officinalis*), promptly to prevent unwanted seedlings germinating all over the garden.

Stocking the herb garden

For a good range of plants you will need to start by buying some in pots from a specialist outlet. For economy, choose small pots, though larger specimens will provide material to cut more quickly. Other herbs are best grown from seed, especially annuals. If you have access to established plants, digging up and dividing clumps of fibrous-rooted herbs, such as marjoram or chives, is a good way to increase stocks as well as rejuvenate existing plants. Some herbs, including houseleek (*Sempervivum tectorum*) and chamomile (*Chamaemelum nobile*) conveniently provide offsets or runners for planting out.

SOWING SEEDS

To give plants an early start and maximize germination, sow seeds in trays, in the spring, under glass. Label the tray with the seed name (all seedlings look very similar when they have just germinated).

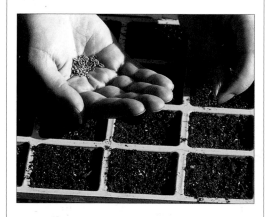

1 Fill a seed tray with soilless compost (growing medium). A tray divided into cells makes it easier to sow the seeds thinly and to pot up seedlings later on. Water the compost first, then scatter two or three seeds in each compartment.

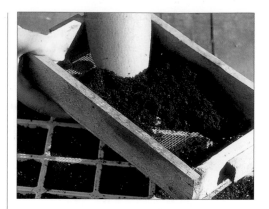

2 Cover the tray with a thin layer of sifted compost. Water again very lightly.

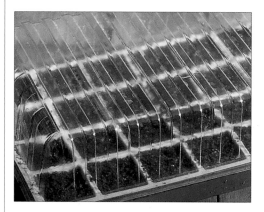

3 Put a polythene (plastic) dome over the tray, or enclose it in a clear plastic bag. Put the tray on a windowsill or in the greenhouse and cover with black polythene until the seedlings begin to show.

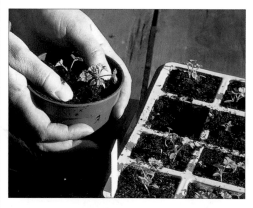

4 When the seedlings come through, remove the cover and keep them moist. As soon as they are large enough to handle, pot them up individually and harden off before planting outside.

PLANTING OFFSETS

Plants such as chamomile (*Chamaemelum nobile*) and houseleek (*Sempervivum tectorum*) send out little satellite plants, or offsets (offshoots), which can be separated and replanted, either directly in the garden or in pots. Replant them in spring.

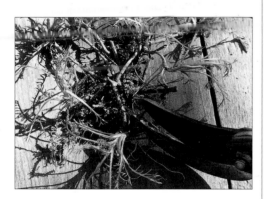

1 Lift a plant (in this case, chamomile) and separate the offsets, making sure each piece has some root attached.

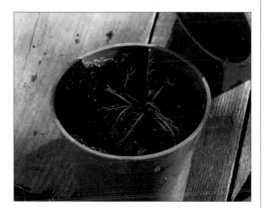

2 Press each new plantlet into a pot of compost (growing medium). Water and leave in a shady place until new roots develop.

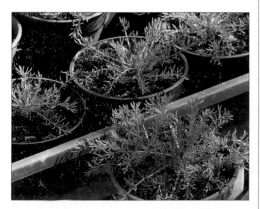

3 The cuttings will grow into bushy plants in 2–3 weeks, when they can be potted on into larger pots or planted out in the garden.

PLANTING A HERB GARDEN

Spring is a good time for planting a herb garden. The ground starts to warm up and the days lengthen, providing optimum growing conditions. Annuals, such as chervil (*Anthriscus cerefolium*) and coriander (*Coriandrum sativum*) (cilantro) are best sown directly where they are to grow. Others, including parsley (*Petroselinum crispum*) and basil (*Ocimum basilicum*), are successful when raised in trays for growing on and setting out later. Half-hardy herbs, such as basil and nasturtium (*Tropaeolum majus*), should not be planted outside until all danger of frost is past.

Shrubby plants like lavender (*Lavandula* spp), and trees, such as elder (*Sambucus nigra*) or bay (*Laurus nobilis*), can also be planted out in autumn. Prepare the ground well first.

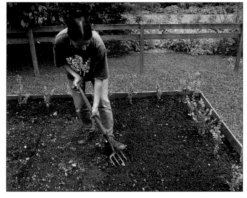

1 Fork over the planting area, removing weeds and breaking up and turning over the soil. Improve very heavy soils by digging in grit and compost to improve drainage. Work the soil to a fine tilth.

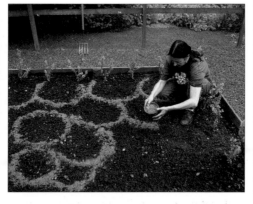

2 Using sand, divide the area into planting bays, allowing sufficient room in each for a plant to spread and grow.

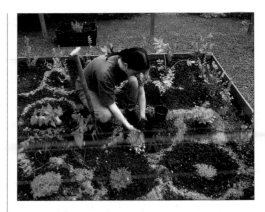

3 Dig a hole in the centre of each area deep enough to plant the herb. Tap the plant out of its container, position it and backfill with soil. Adding compost or organic matter at the planting stage gives plants a good start.

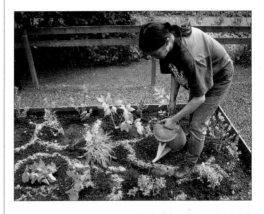

4 Soak plants well in their pots for an hour before setting them out in the garden. Water them again immediately after planting. Keep them well watered until the roots are fully established in the surrounding soil.

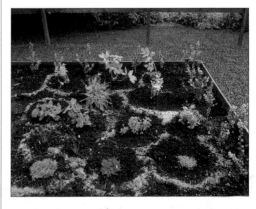

5 Keep the whole area weed free to give the plants a chance to become well established. As they spread and outgrow their space, some of the herbs can be dug up and replanted elsewhere.

Harvesting, Drying and Storing

Growing your own herbs means you can preserve them for later use. This is particularly beneficial during the winter when plants are dormant. Harvesting plants at the right time and drying and storing them carefully will ensure they retain maximum fragrance and medicinal properties for as long as possible.

Harvesting herbs

The various parts of a herb, including the leaves, flowers, fruits and seeds, may be gathered at different times, depending upon the plant and the part that provides the desirable properties. Annual leafy herbs such as basil (*Ocimum basilicum*) and parsley (*Petroselinum crispum*) should be carefully picked, never taking more than about 10 per cent of the growth in a single picking.

The same is true of perennials such as sage (*Salvia officinalis*), thyme (*Thymus vulgaris*) and rosemary (*Rosmarinus officinalis*), because severe pruning or overstripping of the leaves will weaken the plant. It is important that you do not remove more than one-third of the growth at any one time. If you harvest carefully you will get a more vigorous leaf growth that will result in healthier plants.

As a general rule, pick herbs just before the plant is about to flower, which is when the leaves have the strongest flavour. Pick leaves when they are fresh and at their sweetest, selecting blemish-free upper leaves. Collect the leaves in the early morning or evening, provided they are dry, rather than in bright afternoon sun when the plant's sap is rising. The aroma of herbs is at its strongest at this time of day and it is easily lost if picked then. Flowers such as borage (*Borago officinalis*) and lavender (*Lavandula* spp), however, are best picked just before they reach full bloom and once they begin to open in the heat of the day.

Roots and rhizomes, such as black cohosh (*Cimicifuga racemosa*) and echinacea (*E. purpurea*), are collected in autumn, when the maximum amount of nutrition has been stored. Use a fork to tease the roots from the soil; avoid "hand-pulling" them. Choose

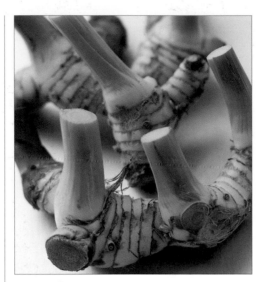

Above *Galangal* (Alpinia officinarum) *root is harvested for use in culinary and herbal preparations.*

the best and use a brush to loosen any dirt. If you need to wash them, avoid soaking as this can leach out active constituents.

Harvesting seeds tends to vary from plant to plant. Some seeds, like those of borage (*Borago officinalis*), fall to the ground as soon as they are ripe. Thyme (*Thymus* spp) seeds are very small and hard to see. Parsley (*Petroselinum crispum*) and coriander (*Coriandrum sativum)* seeds shake off easily, and frequently the plants will have sown next year's crop for you before you realize they have gone to seed. One method of harvesting any seed that is difficult to collect is to tie a small paper bag over the flower head when the seeds start to form, ensuring that you can collect the seed without losing any. Use this method for collecting from plants with small seeds, as they can drop off when ripe or may spring from the plant.

Drying herbs

One of the most popular methods of preserving herbs for use during the winter months is drying. This method may actually improve the flavour of culinary bay leaves (*Laurus nobilis*).

When drying herbs, the temperature of the area should not exceed 30°C/86°F because the plants' essential oils will

evaporate at or above this temperature. Do not dry your herbs in the kitchen where they will be spoiled by steam.

Spread leaves, flowers or petals on newspaper or put small bunches of herbs into brown paper bags. Store them in a dry, dark, warm place until the herbs inside are crumbly, shaking the bags occasionally so that the plants dry evenly. The process should take up to a week. Roots are best chopped into small pieces and dried in a very low oven.

Drying seeds

Collect the seeds just as they are ripening. Remove any chaff or plant debris and spread the seeds out on a tray or in a paper or muslin bag. Leave in a cool, dark place for a few days until the seed is completely dry. Once the seeds have been dried they can be stored in airtight containers, such as dark-coloured glass jars with well-fitting lids. Label the jars with the name of each herb and the date of picking for future reference, and store them in a cool, dry place, protected from light.

Below *Set a space aside for preparing herbs, and keep it clean so that the dried herbs do not become contaminated.*

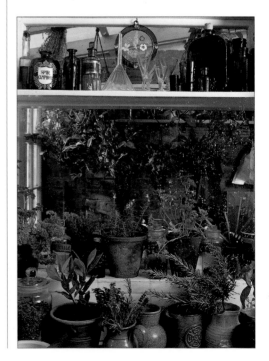

Storing herbs

Rub leafy herbs off their stems once they are dry. The job is easier if you wear light cotton gloves. Dried herbs deteriorate quickly if left out in the light and air, so store them in a cool, dark place in airtight, dark glass or pottery jars. Herbs also keep well in sealed brown paper bags. Cellophane bags are fine for short periods, but do not use polythene (plastic) bags or containers as they draw out residual moisture in the material. Dried herbs should not be exposed to any dampness. If left in unsealed containers, they will take in moisture from the surrounding air.

Although many herbs retain an aromatic scent for several years after drying, it is best to replace stocks every year since their potency declines with age. Drying your own herbs allows you to know exactly how old your stock is.

Other ways of preserving and storing herbs

Although drying is the most common way to preserve leafy herbs for use when fresh are not in season, it is not the only possibility. Other traditional ways of preserving herbs include steeping them in oil or vinegar, or in sugar syrups, all of which take on their flavours. The methods described below are also effective ways of retaining the properties and fragrance of herbs for later use.

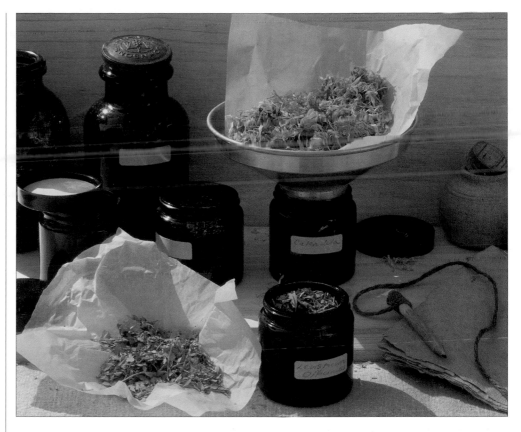

cool oven for 10–20 minutes. When the herbs are dry, let them cool and place in a jar. Chives (*Allium schoenoprasum*), oregano (*Origanum* spp), thyme (*Thymus* spp), lemon balm (*Melissa officinalis*), parsley (*Petroselinum crispum*), rosemary (*Rosmarinus officinalis*) and basil (*Ocimum basilicum*) can all be treated this way.

Above *Store home-dried herbs in dark glass jars to prevent deterioration. Ensure the stock is thoroughly dried and that it is not contaminated with dust. Label the jars with the date and name of the herb.*

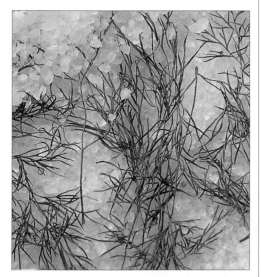

Herb salts (above)

Spread a layer of coarse salt on a sheet of baking parchment. Sprinkle the chopped fresh herbs on top of the salt and bake in a

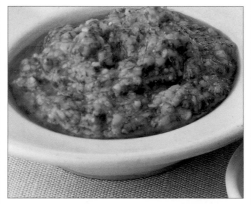

Puréeing (above)

To retain the flavour of fresh basil leaves, mix approximately 60ml/4 tbsp olive oil with 2 cups of the leaves, which have been washed and dried. Blend in a food processor to a smooth purée, then transfer to a jar. Stir each time you use it and top with a thin layer of oil afterwards. The purée should keep for up to one week in a refrigerator.

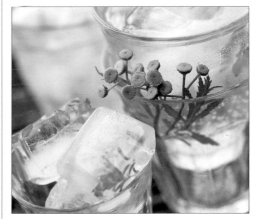

Freezing herbs (above)

Herbs such as dill (*Anethum graveolens*), fennel (*Foeniculum vulgare*), basil and parsley freeze well. The herbs should be cleaned and put into separate, labelled freezer bags. Alternatively, chop the herbs finely and half-fill each compartment of an ice cube tray, then top up with water before freezing. Transfer the frozen cubes to labelled plastic bags and freeze for up to six months. Use in cooking.

Other Herbal Remedy Ingredients

As well as the plants you grow yourself, there are a number of other ingredients you will need for making herbal preparations, some of which you may have to buy.

Dried herbs

As well as the aerial parts (leaves, stems and flowers), these ingredients may include the roots or bark of some species. Although it is useful to dry as many of your own herbs as possible, you will not be able to grow everything you need and there are times when it is more convenient to buy some. Choose a reputable supplier with a high turnover of product, and buy in small quantities, as it is not worthwhile to keep dried herbs at the back of the cupboard for years: use them within 6 months to a year.

Resins

• **Benzoin** is an aromatic resin from the styrax tree. It has preservative and antiseptic properties and is used to treat coughs and to calm the system. It is available as a tincture or in ground form.

• **Frankincense** is the gum resin produced by *Boswellia* spp, a genus of shrubby trees from the Arabian peninsula. It can be bought as grains or powder.

• **Myrrh**, the gum resin of another small tree (*Commiphora myrrha*) from the Middle East and the Horn of Africa, has antifungal and antiseptic properties. It can be bought in the form of a tincture or as grains or powder.

Below Resins can be obtained in block or powdered form.

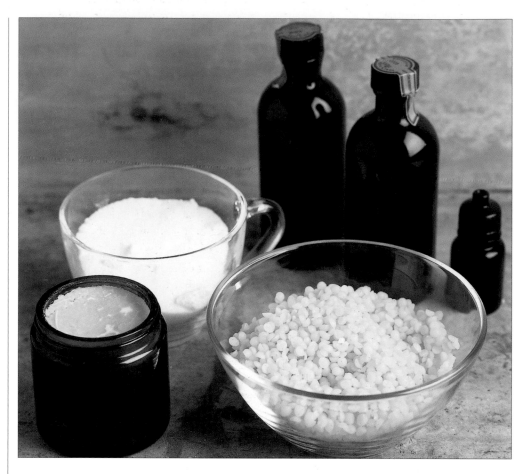

Above Cocoa butter, borax, almond oil, lavender water and beeswax granules.

Powders

• **Slippery elm**, the powdered bark of an elm tree (*Ulmus rubra*) native to North America, has strengthening, healing properties and is used in poultices.

• **Borax** is a mineral deposited on the shores of alkaline lakes. It has cleansing properties and acts as an emulsifier to bind oils and water together. It is toxic if ingested in large quantities, but is safe to use in small amounts in home-made preparations.

• **Fuller's earth** is a clay-like substance, rich in minerals, used to absorb oils. It has good drawing and stimulating properties. It is an ingredient in poultices and face masks.

Below Slippery elm powder is made from the bark of several species of elm tree.

Below Cayenne pepper has antibacterial properties.

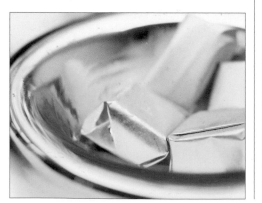

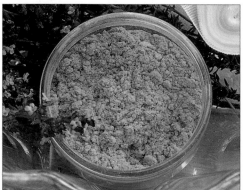

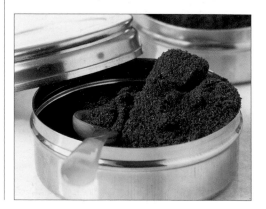

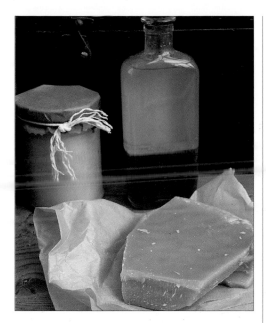

Above *Beeswax is a natural emulsifier and gives creams and ointments a firm texture.*

Spices

• **Cayenne** or chilli pepper stimulates the circulation and increases blood flow. It is harmful in excessive doses.

• **Cinnamon**, made from the rolled bark of a tropical tree (*Cinnamomum* spp), comes as "sticks" or in ground form. It is antibacterial, antifungal and has digestive properties.

• **Cloves** are the dried, immature flower buds of the tree *Syzygium aromaticum*. Stimulating and warming, they are also antiseptic and slightly anaesthetic in action.

• **Ginger** is the rhizome of a tropical plant, *Zingiber officinale*, which can be used fresh

Below *Commercially available herbal tablets may contain additives.*

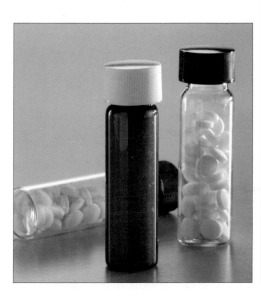

or dried, or in powdered form. It stimulates the circulation and has many uses in home remedies. High doses can be toxic and should be avoided in pregnancy.

• **Mace** and **nutmeg** both come from the fruit of the tree, *Myristica fragrans*. Mace is the outer casing of the fruit and nutmeg is the kernel. Nutmeg is a digestive and helps prevent nausea, but is harmful in large doses. The essential oil of the plant is used in anti-rheumatic remedies.

Oils and waxes

• **Beeswax** is a natural emulsifier for creams and ointments, with a high melting point and stiff texture. It is naturally yellow.

• **Cocoa butter** is the richly moisturizing fat from the cocoa bean.

• **Coconut oil** is extracted from white coconut flesh and is an excellent moisturizer for the skin. Solid at room temperature, it melts when lukewarm.

• **Emulsifying wax** is a petroleum-based wax used for binding oil and water. Although it is not an entirely "natural" product, it makes the best and simplest base for soft-textured home-made creams.

• **Petroleum jelly**, a mineral jelly, is not easily absorbed by the skin and forms a protective layer over it.

Base oils

The best base oils for use in herbal preparations are almond oil, grapeseed oil, sesame oil and jojoba oil. They are used as "carriers" to dilute essential oils.

Below *Essential oils are diluted in a base oil.*

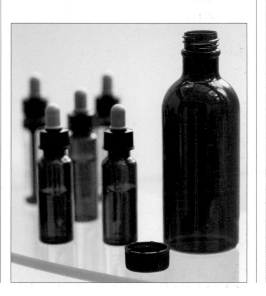

Ready-made remedies

Chosen with care, ready-made products have a valuable place in the home medicine chest.

• **Tinctures**: It is possible to make your own tinctures at home, but it is not easy to obtain all the raw ingredients necessary, and sometimes it is simply more convenient to buy a ready-made product. Manufactured tinctures vary in strength and quality, so read the labels carefully to check the contents and proportions. The proportion of herb material to liquid should be from 1:3 to 1:5, with an alcohol content of 45–50 per cent in water, depending on the herb used. The alcohol is likely to be derived from a source such as sugar beet. Tinctures provide a stronger, more concentrated way of taking a herb than infusions or decoctions. If you dilute the required dose in hot water before taking it, some of the alcohol should evaporate.

• **Herbal fluid extracts**: These are similar to tinctures, but more concentrated. They are obtainable alcohol-free. As they are so much stronger, check the labels carefully and adjust the amount you use accordingly.

• **Capsules**: Usually filled with dried, powdered herbs or a liquid extract, capsules provide a way to take an exactly measured, concentrated dose of a herb and are often standardized for quality. Follow the manufacturer's directions, or consult a qualified herbalist.

• **Tablets**: These may not be such a good choice as capsules, as they are usually made with compressed dried herbs and contain binding agents and often other additives, including artificial sweeteners and colours.

• **Macerated oils**: Herb material is steeped in a vegetable oil (preferably almond oil) to make these products. Although they are similar to the infused oils you can make for yourself, some, such as pot marigold (*Calendula*) and myrrh, are worth buying for convenience, or in order to obtain a stronger or standardized product.

Essential Oils

Essential oils are volatile liquids that are extracted from aromatic plants. They have immense therapeutic value and are often helpful in alleviating the symptoms of ill health in both physical and emotional conditions. They are used in herbal remedies in many different ways, such as diluted in a base oil and applied as a massage to relieve aches and pains, added to infusions to make compresses for sprains or bruises, incorporated into creams and ointments, mixed into decongestant steam inhalations or released into the air by vaporizing them in an essential oil burner to help improve mood.

Despite the name, essential oils are nearer to water in consistency than oil – a drop applied to paper does not usually leave any mark. They are highly volative liquids, which means they evaporate at normal air temperature. It is the essential oil in a plant that gives it its scent and it is secreted in minute glands and hairs in the leaves, stems, flowers, seeds, fruit, roots or bark. Not all plants contain essential oils.

Some plants, such as roses, contain their essential oil mainly in their flowers; others, such as lemon balm (*Melissa officinalis*),

Below *Rose essential oil, distilled from highly fragrant species such as* Rosa mundi, *helps to lift depression and is good for the skin.*

mainly in the leaves. The orange tree (*Citrus aurantium*) contains three differently named essential oils, in the flowers (neroli), the leaves (petitgrain) and the rind of the fruit (orange oil).

The organic chemical structure of plant essential oils is extremely complex. Analysis by gas liquid chromatography reveals that peppermint oil, whose 50 per cent menthol content provides its minty smell, has 98 other constituents. Flower essential oils have as many as several hundred components. For this reason it is impossible to chemically reproduce an exact copy of a naturally occurring essential oil in the laboratory.

Production of essential oils

Essential oils are soluble in fats, vegetable and mineral oils and in alcohol. For the most part they do not dissolve in water, though some of their constituents may do so. The main fragrance molecules of roses and orange flowers, for example, are soluble in water. Steam distillation is the most frequent method of extraction, and volatile solvents and alcohol are sometimes used in the process. A few fragile flower fragrances are still obtained by the centuries-old method of "enfleurage" – macerating the petals in trays of fat – and volatile oil from orange rind is extracted by expression: that is by pressing it

out, now by machine, but formerly by hand. Quality is affected by varying soils, climates and harvesting conditions. Some oils may be diluted or adulterated, and it is not easy to tell, so look for a reliable source.

Essential oils in history

Plant essential oils take their name from the *quinta essentia*, or quintessence, a term coined by the Swiss physician Paracelsus, (1493–1541). He took the medieval theory of alchemy, which sought to isolate the *prima materia*, or elemental matter, of a substance, and applied it specifically to plants, to divide the "essential matter" of a plant from its "non-essential" components.

In ancient times, extracting plant fragrance by macerating it in oil or fat was common, and a technique of destructive distillation, such as that which produces oil of turpentine, was also known. At the beginning of the 11th century, steam distillation was discovered as a means of making plant-scented waters. It is usually credited to the Persian scholar and physician Avicenna, author of *The Canon of Medicine*. Arnald de Villanova, a Spanish physician

Below *Use a vegetable oil, such as almond, as a base oil for massage, to enable the essential oils to be absorbed by the skin.*

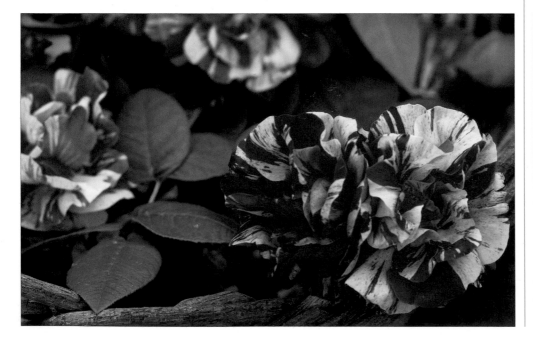

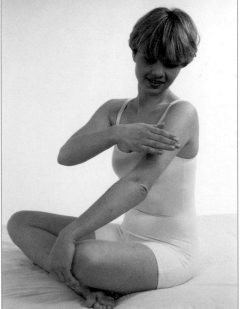

who died in 1311, popularized the use of distilled herb waters for medicinal purposes.

Distillation was seen at the time as a means of refining plant material to its purest form, through fire, and alcohol was widely used in the process because it was considered to produce the best results. It was not until the mid-16th century that the nature of essential oils was understood and the process of separating them from the distillate was put into practice.

By the beginning of the 17th century plant essential oils were available from professional pharmacies, as well as being produced on a domestic scale. Herbals and recipe books contained detailed instructions.

The power of plant fragrances

Fragrances have been revealed by many research studies to have powerful psychological effects. Some fragrances have a calming influence and others are stimulating. One six-month hospital trial found that diffusing lavender oil at night helped elderly patients to sleep better, and in Japan citrus and woody aromas are piped into offices to keep workers alert.

As well as elevating mood or acting as an aid to meditation, vaporizing plant essential oils, so that the scent molecules are dispersed through the air, has other practical benefits. Some, including tea tree, pine and eucalyptus, can destroy airborne bacteria; others, such as peppermint or lemongrass, have insect-repellent properties.

It is often claimed by scientists that synthetic plant scents are indistinguishable from natural ones, but a laboratory-made version of an essential oil replicates only its main components, perhaps five or six out of a total of more than a hundred, and cannot possibly have the same therapeutic powers.

Phototoxic oils

Most citrus oils, especially bergamot oil, make the skin more sensitive to sunlight; you should not apply them to the skin shortly before going in the sun or using a sunbed as they may cause alterations to your skin's pigmentation. It is possible to buy citrus oils that have had the offending ingredient (bergaptene) removed, but there is some question as to whether this reduces the efficacy of the oil. These treated oils are also

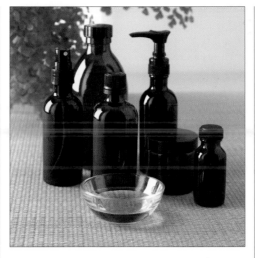

Above *Two or three essential oils can be combined to make effective blends.*

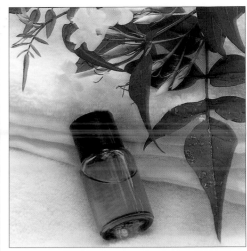

Above *Essential oil of jasmine is obtained by enfleurage, which uses fat to capture the fragrant compounds in the flowers.*

much more expensive. You should retain a sense of proportion about this: perfumes are also phototoxic and should not be worn when sunbathing, as they can cause Berloque dermatitis, an irritating skin rash.

Buying essential oils

Choosing a good quality oil is not easy. You can be sure of its molecular structure and constituents only by having it analysed in a laboratory. It helps to:
• Find a reputable supplier.
• Check the price, especially for rose and

other oils that are expensive to produce. Adulterated or inferior oils may be too cheap for what they purport to be.
• Look at the label – it should say "pure essential oil", not "herbal oil", which means it could be diluted in vegetable oil.
• Check that the label shows the full botanic name of the plant.

Below *A wooden box is ideal for storing a collection of essential oils, as it will protect them from the damaging effects of light.*

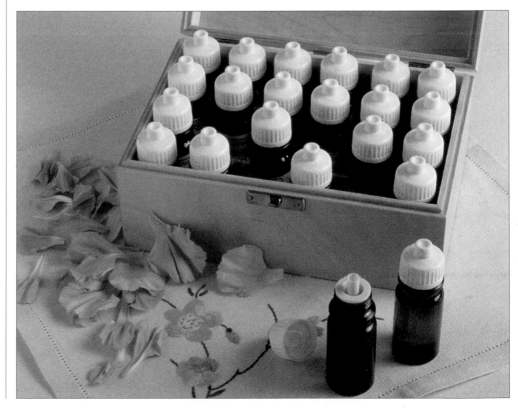

Aromatherapy

The term "aromatherapy" was coined in the early 20th century by a French chemist, René Maurice Gattefossé, who worked in his family's perfumery business. He found that essential oils are absorbed by the body from 30 minutes to 12 hours after being rubbed on to the skin, and he was among the first to recognize the therapeutic effects of essential oils. Another founder was Jean Valnet, a French army surgeon who used essential oils to good effect on the wounds of soldiers during World War II.

The concept of aromatherapy was introduced to Britain as a beauty therapy in the 1950s by Marguerite Maury, who was married to a French doctor and homeopath. It later spread to many other countries around the globe and is now widely recognized as a viable alternative therapy, with its positive benefits even acknowledged by many in the orthodox medical profession.

The healing power of fragrance has a long history, and modern research studies have confirmed its influence over mood and emotion. Essential oils are especially useful for ailments connected with the nervous system and are helpful, for example, in cases of mild depression or when feeling low.

But they have many other uses. The dividing line between aromatherapy and herbal medicine is a slim one, in the sense that essential oils have a place in many herbal home remedies. Their main applications are in massage oils, vaporizers, creams and ointments, or added to baths, foot baths, compresses and steam inhalations. They should not be taken internally without professional advice.

A MASSAGE BLEND

Vegetable oils are excellent carriers for massage. Essential oils readily dissolve in them, and they allow the hands to move continuously on the skin without dragging or slipping. Mineral oil, such as baby oil, aims to protect the skin by keeping moisture out and will not allow essential oils to penetrate, so it is not a suitable oil base. Care should be taken not to use too much of the mixed oil as it can stain sheets and

clothes. To stop too much oil coming out at a time, place your fingers over the top of the bottle, tipping it against them.

Ingredients

15–20 drops essential oil (one oil or a combination of 2–3 oils of your choice)
50ml/2fl oz almond oil

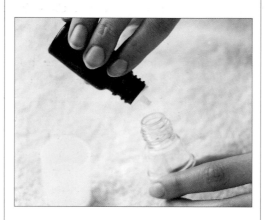

1 Measure your chosen essential oil or oils into a 50ml/2fl oz bottle. (To make a smaller amount, use a total of 8 drops in 25ml/1fl oz base oil, or 1–2 drops in 5ml/1 tsp base oil).

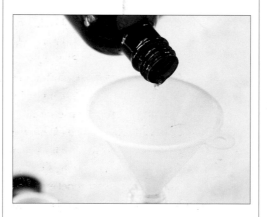

2 Fill the bottle containing the essential oil drops almost to the top with almond oil. Use a funnel, if necessary, to avoid any spillage.

3 Screw on the top securely and label the bottle with the quantity of each oil used, what the mixture is to be used for, your name and the date. Store all essential oils in a cool dark place away from direct sunlight to stop the quality deteriorating.

Safe use of essential oils

Essential oils are very powerful and should always be used sparingly. Doubling the recommended quantities will do more harm than good.

• Do not take essential oils internally without advice and guidance from a qualified aromatherapist.

• Store oils out of reach of children, in a cool, dark cupboard. When you first use an essential oil, it is sensible to do a patch test if you have reactive skin or a tendency to allergies or asthma. Mix 2 drops of essential oil with 5ml/1 tsp almond oil and apply a little to the inner arm or wrist (where skin is most sensitive). Leave for 24 hours without washing the area. If no redness or irritation develops the oil is safe to use.

• Oils should not be used undiluted – the only exception is lavender oil, which can be used on minor cuts or burns. Others must be mixed with a "base" or "carrier" oil before being applied to the skin, or they will cause irritation: in this book, almond oil is the base oil for most projects using essential oils.

• Anyone with a serious medical condition should not use essential oils without consulting their medical practicitioner and, even then, should use them only with the assistance of a qualified aromatherapist.

• Certain essential oils should not be handled by anyone who is or may be pregnant. These include cedarwood, chamomile, clary sage, frankincense, basil, jasmine, marjoram, peppermint and rosemary.

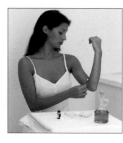

Left *Before using oils test them on a small patch of skin and leave to see if there is a reaction.*

Healing oils for home treatments

Here are some of the therapeutic properties of popular essential oils. Not all these oils will be suitable for everyone. Check the safety of any oil you use, particularly for someone who suffers from a chronic condition such as high blood pressure, or who is pregnant. Some men do not like flowery scents, but these can be combined with a citrus or woody oil to make them acceptable.

Oil	Description	Uses
• Bergamot	A flowery aroma	Antiseptic and pain-relieving; uplifting antidepressant. A good insect repellent and helpful for skin problems. Do not sunbathe for 12 hours after application.
• Chamomile	Blue oil with a gentle apple-like aroma	German chamomile relieves blisters and inflammation; Roman chamomile helps promote restful sleep and soothes aches and skin conditions.
• Frankincense	The aroma of camphor with a hint of lemon	Calms anxiety and has an uplifting effect. May relieve heavy periods. Good for mature skin and also has antiseptic properties.
• Ginger	Sweet, woody aroma	Warming: helps with aches, pains and sports injuries, arthritis, muscle spasm and poor circulation. Aids digestion and helps with travel sickness.
• Grapefruit	Tangy aroma that mixes well with flowery oils	Uplifting and works as an antidepressant. A good cleansing oil. Can help boost the immune system.
• Jasmine	Floral, slightly heady fragrance	Excellent for anxiety and menstrual problems. Considered an aphrodisiac. May be helpful in labour.
• Lavender	Slightly mossy, woody scent	Suitable for stress-related or nervous conditions. It has anti-inflammatory, antiseptic properties, and can help with skin problems and healing.
• Lemon	Sharp citrus scent that combines well with heavy floral oils	Helps aches, pains, depression, fluid retention, sluggish circulation and varicose veins. Astringent.
• Mandarin	Faintly orange aroma	Both calming and uplifting; good for anxiety, stress, insomnia and PMS. Often recommended during pregnancy.
• Neroli	Sweet floral scent with a seaweed-like note	Good for depression, shock, exhaustion and insomnia. May improve appearance of broken veins and scar tissue. Can cause drowsiness.
• Peppermint	Strong fresh minty aroma	Stimulates the circulation. Good for hot, aching feet. May cause skin reaction if overused; should not be used for people with epilepsy.
• Rose	Rich floral fragrance	Good for the skin, and may help varicose and broken veins. Helps female complaints such as PMS, as well as grief, depression and fatigue.
• Rosemary	Refreshing camphorous aroma	Soothes aches, pains, stiff muscles, increases alertness, relieves stress and exhaustion. Do not use if you have high blood pressure or epilepsy.
• Sandalwood	Warm, woody smell	Relaxing oil, with antiseptic and anti-inflammatory qualities. Good for dry skin. Helps stress and exhaustion. Said to be an aphrodisiac.
• Tangerine	Tangy, slightly sweet smell	Antispasmodic, helpful for pre-menstrual tension.
• Tea tree	Balsamic aroma	Good first-aid oil for the skin; antifungal, antiviral, anti-inflammatory. Good as an insect repellent; soothes insect bites.
• Thyme	Strong herbal scent	Antiseptic, antispasmodic, antifungal, antiviral. Stimulating oil that boosts concentration. Do not use on sensitive skin.
• Violet	Rich sweet floral	Encourages good circulation and feeds the skin. Pain-relieving and anti-inflammatory properties.
• Ylang-ylang	Powerful spicy scent	Eases tension, stress and fatigue. Over-use can cause headache or irritation.

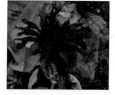
Bergamot

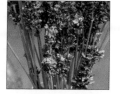
Lavender

Chamomile

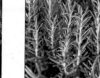
Rosemary

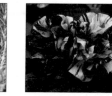
Rose

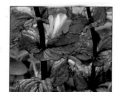
Peppermint

Making Infusions

Many of the active constituents of herbs are soluble in water, and one of the easiest ways to benefit from a herb's properties is to drink it as a tea or infusion. In principle, herb teas are made just like ordinary tea, by pouring hot water over plant material and leaving it to infuse for a short period before straining and drinking it. Many commercial brands are available, usually in the form of teabags, but the taste of teas made from fresh or home-dried garden herbs is hard to beat and ensures maximum benefit from the properties of the plant.

Herbal infusions are also useful in a number of other preparations, from creams to compresses. For these purposes they can be made a little stronger by increasing the quantity of herbs by up to one-third and leaving them to infuse a little longer. Herbal infusions for use in such preparations can be left to cool, stored in the refrigerator and used within 24 hours.

What herbs to use
Herb teas are usually made from the aerial parts of the plant: these are the leaves, stems or flowers, as appropriate. They can be used fresh or dried. Fresh herbs, such as rosemary, lemon balm and lemon verbena, provide a pleasant, lively taste, but dried herbs may sometimes be more convenient to use, especially in the winter when stocks are low.

Herbs vary in potency and when making them into teas, you will need less of a strong-tasting herb than one with a weaker flavour.

As a general rule you need twice as much fresh plant material as dried. This is because the water content has been removed from dried herbs, making them stronger and less bulky. Dried herbs that are loosely cut, or left whole (such as lemon verbena (*Aloysia triphylla*)) are bulkier than if finely cut or powdered.

When making any herbal preparation from fresh material, correct identification of the plant you are using is crucial. If in doubt, do not use the plant.

A FRESH HERB TEA
Leafy fresh herbs cannot be measured by volume as they are too bulky, so they must be weighed. Wash them before use, especially if they have been picked from the wild. A cafétière is convenient, but you can also use an ordinary teapot or a jug with a lid, then strain the tea into a cup to drink. For a single cup, use 10g/⅓oz fresh herb (or two small sprigs).

Ingredients
30g/1oz fresh herb
600ml/1pint/2½ cups boiling water

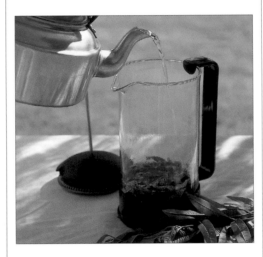

1 Warm the cafétière or pot and put in the herbs. Pour on boiling water and replace the lid to prevent the vapour dissipating.

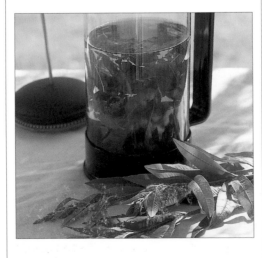

2 Leave to brew for 3–4 minutes, then depress the plunger or strain the tea into a cup for a refreshing drink.

A DRIED HERB TEA
When finely cut or powdered, dried herbs can be measured by volume, in the same way that you would measure out coffee. But when they are bulky, loose-cut leaves, such as home-dried lemon verbena (*Aloysia triphylla*), it is not possible to measure them in a spoon, and they must be weighed.

Ingredients
15ml/1tbsp finely cut dried herb, or
15g/½oz loose-cut dried herb
600ml/1pt/2½ cups boiling water

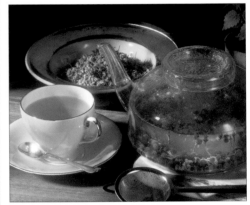

Make the infusion in the same way as for fresh herb tea. For a single cup use 5ml/1 tsp finely cut herb, or 5g/⅙oz loose-cut dried herb.

Below *A tea infuser is useful for making a herbal infusion in an individual cup, and saves having to strain out the herb.*

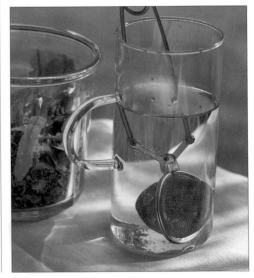

Making Decoctions and Syrups

Infusing in boiling water works well with the aerial parts of herbs, but is not enough to extract the active constituents from roots or bark, the parts used in herbs such as valerian (*Valeriana officinalis*), ginger (*Zingiber officinale*) and cramp bark (*Viburnum opulus*). This harder plant material needs to be simmered in water. The resulting liquid is strained off and is called a decoction.

MAKING A DECOCTION

Decoctions are used for similar purposes as herbal infusions: they can be taken internally to relieve a variety of conditions, such as cold symptoms, or applied externally as lotions or compresses.

Ingredients

30g/1oz herb material (roots, rhizomes or
    bark), freshly harvested or dried
1 litre/1½ pints/3¾ cups water

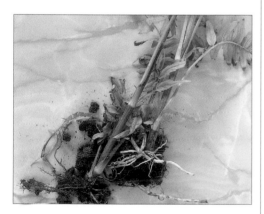

1 Roots and barks need to be prepared for use when harvested in the autumn.

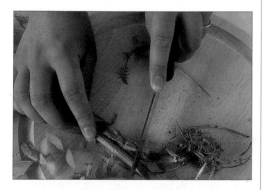

2 Trim the aerial parts of the plant away from the root.

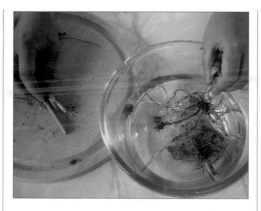

3 Wash the roots thoroughly in clean water, then chop into small pieces.

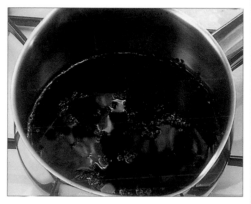

4 Put 30g/1oz of the herb material into a pan (not aluminium), and add the water. Bring to the boil and simmer for 15–20 minutes or until the liquid has reduced to 600ml/1pt/2½ cups. Remove from the heat.

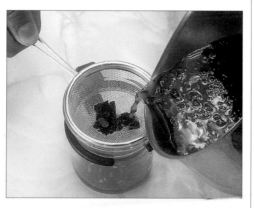

5 Strain the liquid and allow to cool before drinking, or cover and chill for to 24 hours. Decoctions can be drunk hot or cold. They can also be used as ingredients in other herbal products.

MAKING A SYRUP

Herb syrups conserve the active constituents of plants and are useful for preserving items such as elderberries for winter coughs and colds. A syrup is also a useful way to improve the flavour of bitter herbs such as mugwort (*Artemisia vulgaris*) and vervain (*Verbena officinalis*).

Ingredients

500g/1¼lb sugar or honey
1¾ pints/4 cups water
150g/5oz plant material

1 Place the sugar or honey in a pan. Add the water. Heat gently, stirring, to dissolve. Add the herbs and heat gently for 5 minutes.

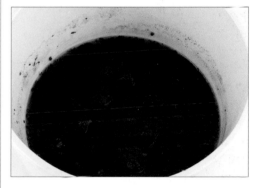

2 Turn off the heat and allow to steep overnight. Strain and store in a sterilized airtight container in the refrigerator.

Below *Syrups will keep for 18 months.*

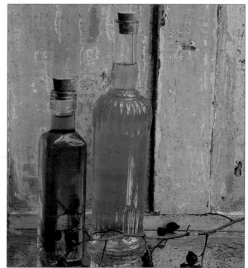

Making Tinctures

A tincture provides a more concentrated herbal product than either an infusion or a decoction. It is made by steeping the prepared herb material in a mixture of alcohol and water for several weeks: this extracts both the non-water-soluble and water-soluble active constituents.

Fresh or dried herb material can be used to make tinctures. Leaves, stems, flowers, berries, even roots, may all be suitable, depending on the plant.

Storing tinctures

The alcohol used to steep the herbs acts as a preservative, so tinctures will keep for up to 2 years. Strain them into sterilized dark glass bottles with tight-fitting stoppers to prevent deterioration of the contents. If you do need to use clear glass, keep the tinctures in a dark cupboard to protect them from light.

A TINCTURE

Useful tinctures include lavender for headaches, raspberry leaf for mouth ulcers, elderflower for colds, juniper for rheumatism, and sweet violet for insomnia. Vodka is the most appropriate alcohol for home-made tinctures, since it is a pure spirit containing few additives. In order to make the tincture strong enough, the herb material has to be soaked in the alcohol and water in batches, as there is not enough liquid to cover all the herbs at once.

Ingredients

100g/4oz dried herbs or 300g/
    11oz fresh herbs
250ml/8fl oz/1 cup vodka
100ml/4fl oz water

CAUTION Under no circumstances use industrial alcohol or white spirits to make tinctures, as they are highly toxic.

Right *Tinctures are an effective way to extract the active ingredients of plants and are easy to prepare. They can be used in compresses and lotions or diluted and taken internally for various conditions.*

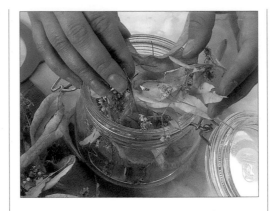

1 Place one third of the given quantity of dried or fresh herbs in a jar.

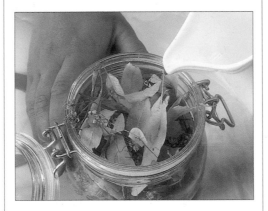

2 Stir the alcohol and water together and pour the mixture over the herbs. Leave the herbs to steep in the liquid for one week, preferably in a warm, dry place.

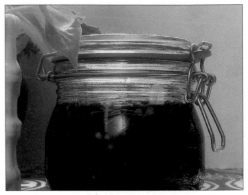

3 Gently shake the jar once a day.

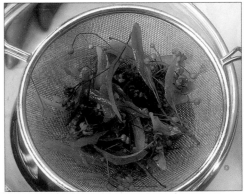

4 Strain and discard the herbs. Substitute a fresh batch and leave for a further week. Repeat with the final batch of herbs, before straining and storing the liquid in a cool dark place.

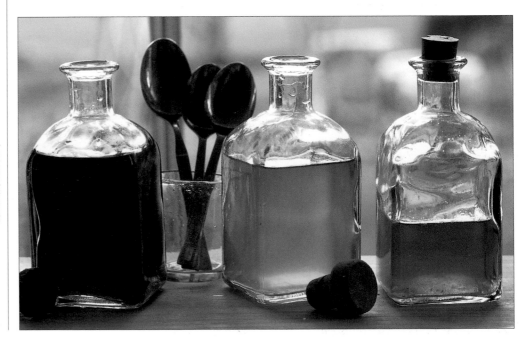

Making Cold-infused Oils

Cold infused oils, also known as "macerated oils" or herbal oils, are simple to prepare and are an effective way to infuse herb material in a vegetable oil base. They are suitable for external use in massage, as bath oils or for conditioning the hair and skin.

It pays to use a good quality oil for massage and therapeutic purposes – such as almond or grapeseed. Sunflower oil can be used, but is more suitable as a culinary oil. It is best not to leave any of the fresh herb in the oil once the infusion is complete, as after a couple of weeks it will start to decay and adversely affect the keeping properties of the oil.

Which herbs to use

Fresh herbs are best for this purpose, but dried ones may also be used. Delicate flower heads, such as chamomile (*Chamaemelum nobile*), marigold (*Calendula officinalis*) or St John's wort (*Hypericum perforatum*), work well, as does more robust herb material, including rosemary, marjoram, thyme, sage and lavender, garlic and spices.

Exact quantities cannot be specified, as the method depends on covering plant material with oil and, depending on which herb you use, you may need to steep several batches in the oil to suffuse it sufficiently with the desired fragrance.

Do not put St John's wort oil directly on to the skin before going out into bright sunlight as it can cause a reaction.

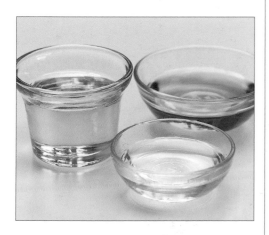

Above *Almond and grapeseed oils are best when making herbal oils for massage.*

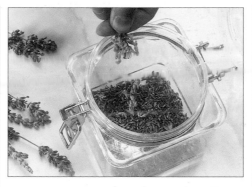

1 Fill a glass storage jar with the flowers or leaves of your chosen herb.

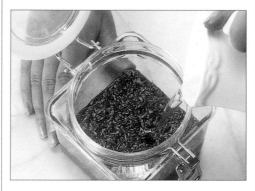

2 Pour in a light vegetable oil to cover the herbs – try sunflower or grapeseed oil.

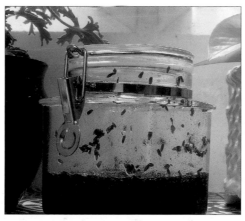

3 Leave the jar to stand on a sunny windowsill for a month to steep. Give it a shake every day.

Right *Massaging the head and hair with herbal oils relieves stress and conditions the scalp at the same time. Ensure that there is time to relax after the massage to fully feel the benefit of it.*

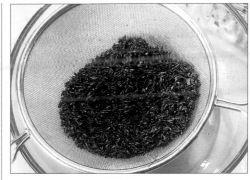

4 Strain the flowers or leaves and discard them. For a stronger infusion, renew the herbs in the oil every 2 weeks.

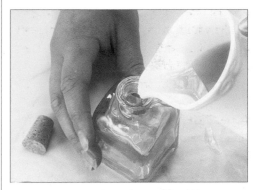

5 Pour the finished infused oil into sterilized stoppered bottles and keep in a dark, dry place for up to 6 months.

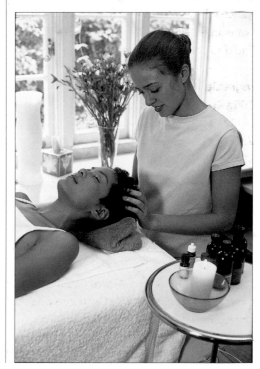

Making Poultices and Compresses

Poultices are made with solid herb material and compresses with liquid preparations. They are applied to the area to be treated using gauze bandaging, or a similar soft material. Both poultices and compresses are helpful in easing general aches and pains, including headache, backache, stomach and period pain, stiff muscles, joint pains and strains, as well as relieving spots, boils, itchy skin and insect bites. They may be used cold or hot, according to the condition being treated.

A HERBAL POULTICE

A poultice is made using the fresh herb applied to the skin at the point of pain or injury and held in place with a bandage. Dried leaves can also be used for convenience, or when no fresh material is available.

Ingredients
handful of fresh herbs or
    30–45ml/2–3 tbsp of dried herbs
boiling water to cover

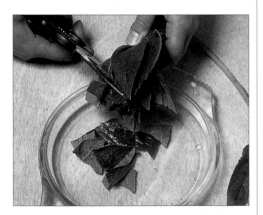

1 Place a handful of roughly chopped clean and freshly picked herb leaves in a bowl and cover with boiling water. Leave to stand for 5–10 minutes. Mash with a fork.

> **CAUTION** Do not use herbal poultices or compresses on broken skin. They may exacerbate the problem.

Right *Essential oils can be used to soak fabric to make a compress or a poultice.*

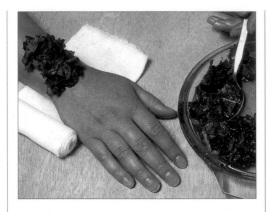

2 Squeeze out the excess liquid and apply the herbs directly to the skin, or place between two layers of gauze. Bind the herbs loosely with a bandage to hold it in place.

A HERBAL COMPRESS

A compress is made by soaking a piece of fabric in a liquid herbal preparation and applying it to the skin of the affected area. For a cold compress, place a sealed plastic bag of frozen vegetables or crushed ice cubes wrapped in fabric over the treatment area and hold in place. For a warm compress, wring out a pad or cloth in the hot liquid and hold it on the area until it cools, then repeat as necessary.

Ingredients
handful of fresh herbs or
    30–45ml/2–3 tbsp dried herbs
    or 2–3 tsp/10–15ml tincture
    or 5–8 drops essential oil
600ml/1pt/2½ cups boiling water

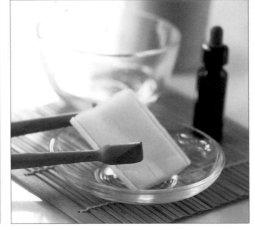

1 To make a herbal infusion, put the fresh or dried herbs in a bowl and pour over the measured amount of boiling water. Leave to stand for 30 minutes to one hour. Alternatively, dilute the herbal tincture or essential oil in hot or cold water.

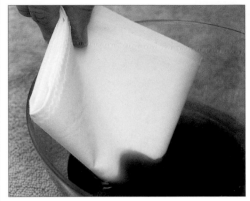

2 Fold a piece of clean, soft cotton fabric into a loose pad, and soak it in the infusion, diluted tincture or essential oil. Wring out the excess liquid.

3 Apply the pad directly to the affected area, holding it in place and repeating as necessary.

Below *A hot compress soothes aching joints and muscles.*

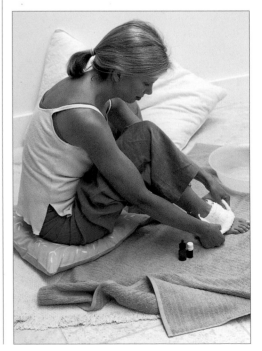

Making Creams and Ointments

Herbal creams and ointments have many uses for soothing and conditioning the skin, or as liniments and rubs for aches and pains.

Though both are used in similar ways their composition is different. A cream is a mixture of oils or fats with water, which softens on the skin and is absorbed into it. An ointment is made of oils or fats but contains no water and is not intended to be absorbed into the skin; instead it provides a barrier or protective layer over it, keeping out dirt and moisture and helping to retain the skin's natural oils.

Making your own creams and ointments is not difficult. You can also buy simple, unperfumed base creams or lotions, to which you can add essential oils, herbs or herbal tinctures as appropriate.

Whether you buy ready-made base creams or make your own, the addition of any plant material, including essential oils and tinctures, will shorten the shelf life of the products and most should be used within 2–3 months.

A HERBAL OINTMENT

Protective barrier ointments were once made from animal fats, but petroleum jelly or paraffin wax makes a longer-lasting base that is more pleasant to apply.

Ingredients
200g/7oz petroleum jelly
30g/1oz fresh herbs, finely chopped, or
    15g/½oz dried herbs

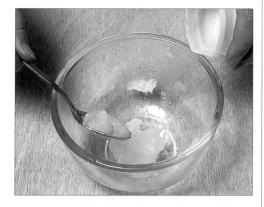

1 Put the petroleum jelly into a bowl and set it over a pan of simmering water to melt.

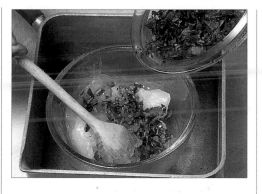

2 Stir in the chopped fresh or dried herbs and continue to heat gently over simmering water, stirring occasionally, for about 1 hour. Strain the mixture through muslin (cheesecloth) or a jelly bag, and pour into a sterilized jar immediately. Seal and label.

CAUTION Do not add more herbal content, essential oil or tincture than specified.

A HERBAL CREAM

Skin creams made from natural ingredients have many uses and are soothing and moisturizing. If you are using essential oils instead of an infusion, lavender, rose and neroli have beneficial properties, and smell delicious. Emulsifying ointment, a product that readily mixes with water, is available from pharmacies and is the standard base for home-made skin creams. It is easy to use and provides the right texture, though it is not an entirely natural product. Natural ingredients that can be used to make creams in the same way include beeswax, coconut oil and cocoa butter, and they are used in some of the recipes for beauty treatments later in this book.

Ingredients
300ml/½ pint/1¼ cups water
30g/1oz fresh herbs or 15g/½oz dried herbs
    or 5–6 drops essential oil
    or 5ml/1 tsp herbal tincture
60ml/4 tbsp emulsifying ointment
15ml/1 tbsp glycerine

Right *Herbal creams should be used soon after making.*

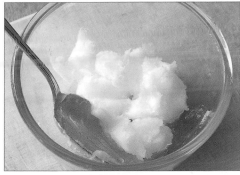

1 Boil the water and pour it over the fresh or dried herbs. Leave to infuse until cool, then strain. Place the emulsifying ointment with the glycerine in a bowl and set it over a pan of simmering water. Heat gently, stirring, until the ointment has melted, then remove the bowl from the heat.

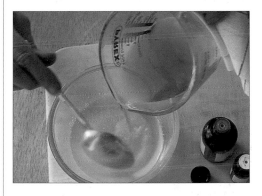

2 Add the cooled herbal infusion (or 300ml/½ pint/1¼ cups plain water to which you have added the essential oil or herbal tincture), and stir until the mixture starts to thicken. Before it has set completely, pour it into a small sterilized jar. Seal, date and label. Keep the cream in a cool place and use it within 2 months.

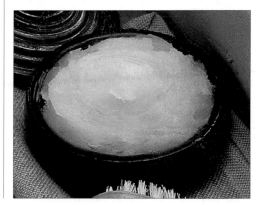

Making Inhalations

Breathing in herbal vapours can be beneficial both for physical and mental conditions. Steam inhalations are an effective way of bringing temporary relief for catarrh and blocked sinuses, and can also be used in facial beauty treatments to open the pores and cleanse the skin. Inhaling just the fragrance of plant essential oils has a powerful effect on mood and mental states. It is simple to do using a vaporizer or essential oil burner to scent the air, which works more subtly than breathing in steam.

A STEAM INHALATION

This old-fashioned treatment remains highly effective as a decongestant. You can use an appropriate essential oil or strong herbal infusion to scent the steaming water, but for the gentlest effect use the fresh herbs themselves.

Ingredients
600ml/1pt/2½ cups water
large handful of fresh herbs
    or 200ml/7fl oz/1 cup strong herbal
    infusion made from fresh or dried herbs
    or 6–8 drops essential oil

1 Boil the water, pour it into a bowl and add the herb material appropriate to the condition you are treating. Add a little cold water.

2 Lean over the bowl, place a towel over both your head and the bowl to retain the steam and aroma, and inhale the steam for a few seconds at a time. Continue for up to 10 minutes overall.

Below *Inhaling steam infused with herbs helps to clear the nasal passages. Allow the water to cool sufficiently first.*

AN ESSENTIAL OIL BURNER

Breathing in essential oil vapours can be relaxing, restorative or uplifting. One way to inhale the scent is simply to put a few drops on a handkerchief and keep it on your pillow overnight. But for a more controlled and concentrated method, which is also longer lasting, an essential oil burner is the answer.

There is a wide range of styles to choose from, but they all work by heating the essential oil in water so that it vaporizes as steam, which can be inhaled. The heat is usually supplied by any candle or nightlight (tealight). Always treat an essential oil burner as you would a candle: do not leave it unattended or with an unsupervised child, and never leave one burning overnight.

Put 6–8 drops of essential oil into the filled water chamber of the burner. Top up the water as it evaporates, adding another 1–2 drops of oil as necessary. A few drops of oil in a bowl of hot water will also scent a room.

CAUTION If you have either high blood pressure or asthma you should seek medical advice before using steam, and in any case do not overdo an inhalation.

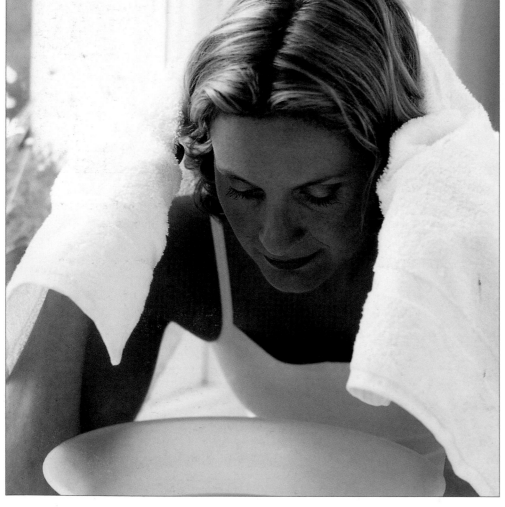

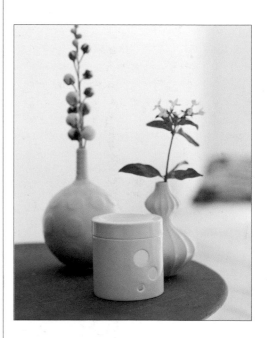

Above *An essential oil burner is a good way to inhale beneficial vapours.*

Making Bath Mixes and Sleep Pillows

Other ways to benefit from the scent of herbs include putting them into bath bags to hang over the taps, allowing the warm water to release a restorative, relaxing steam, or adding them to sleep pillows to help induce a restful night.

A HERBAL BATH MIX

• **Relaxing:** Chamomile (*Chamaemelum nobile*) flowers and foliage.

• **Revitalizing:** Rosemary (*Rosmarinus officinale*), peppermint (*Mentha* x *piperita*), lemon thyme (*Thymus* x *citriodorus*), pine needles.

• **To improve circulation:** Nettles (*Urtica dioica*). These will lose their sting once they have been soaked in hot water.

• **For aches and pains:** Comfrey leaves (*Symphytum officinale*) with 15ml/1 tbsp powdered ginger (*Zingiber officinale*).

• **For colds:** Lavender (*Lavandula*), thyme and a 2.5cm/1in piece of grated fresh ginger.

• **For itchy skin:** Comfrey, houseleek (*Sempervivum tectorum*), lady's mantle (*Alchemilla mollis*), marshmallow (*Althaea officinalis*). Add a cup of cider vinegar to the bath as well.

Below *For a restorative, invigorating bath, hang a herb-filled bath bag over the tap while the water is running, then stir 1kg/2¼lb sea salt into the bath. Soak in it for 10 minutes before scrubbing the skin with the bath bag, to which you have added some grated soap. Finish with a cool shower to leave the skin feeling soft and refreshed.*

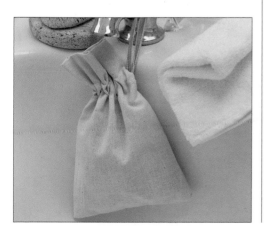

A SLEEP PILLOW

To fill this pillow use a mixed rose pot-pourri incorporating sleep-inducing herbs such as hops (*Humulus lupulus*), chamomile and lavender. Alternatively fill with hops alone.

You will need
40 x 25cm/16 x 10in cotton
 wadding (batting)
pins
sewing machine
matching sewing thread and needle
rose and herb pot-pourri
2 pieces of fabric, 24 x 29cm/9½ x 11½in
1m/1yd gathered broderie anglaise edging
tacking (basting) thread
22cm/8½in strip self-adhesive fabric tape

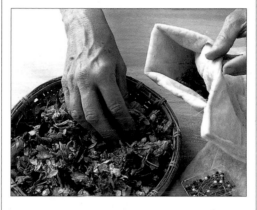

1 To make the inner pad, fold the wadding (batting) in half with the shorter edges together. Pin, then stitch together, leaving an opening at one end. Turn through and fill with pot-pourri. Slip-stitch the opening.

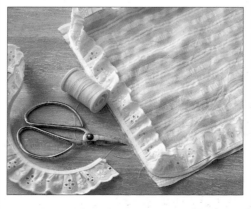

2 To make the decoration on the outer casing, place one cover piece right side up

on a flat surface. Pin and baste the broderie anglaise all around the edge, with the frill facing inwards.

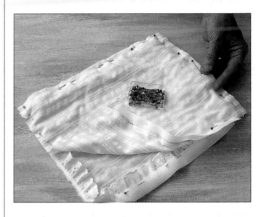

3 Separate the fabric tape and centre the two strips on matching edges of the right side of two cover pieces. Stitch in place. Stitch the covers together around the remaining sides.

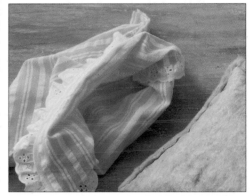

4 Turn the cover through and insert the filled pad. Fasten the fabric tape.

Below *Herbal pillows can aid sleep.*

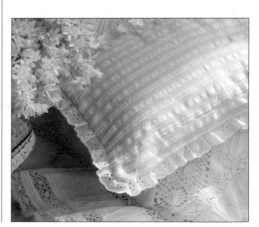

Healing Herbs in Food

There are many health benefits to be gained from adding plenty of herbs to food. Herbs add interest and flavour to bland foods, and are rich in vitamins and minerals: although it may be argued that they are only used in small amounts in many dishes, the effect is cumulative. In some dishes, where a specific herb is the main ingredient – such as basil in pesto sauce or nettles in soup – it will be eaten in more than adequate amounts. Some herb seeds aid digestion and certain familiar food items, such as garlic and oats, have useful herbal applications. Spices are also valuable in the diet for their medicinal properties as well as for flavour.

Reducing fat and salt in the diet

There is no doubt that fat makes food more palatable, and it is all too easy to acquire a taste for over-salty food, but excess salt in the diet has been linked to high blood pressure. If you are trying to cut down on your intake of fat and salt, herb and spice seasonings are a healthy alternative way to add extra flavour to food. Mix dried herbs into soups and casseroles, stir-fries and pasta sauces, or sprinkle them over lightly cooked vegetables. Nothing beats fresh herbs as seasoning. Tie them in small mixed bunches and use as required as a bouquet garni.

Herbs to use in place of salt

- Bay (*Laurus nobilis*)
- Coriander (*Coriandrum sativum*)
- Hyssop (*Hyssopus officinalis*)
- Lovage (*Levisticum officinale*)
- Pot marjoram (*Origanum onites*)
- Rosemary (*Rosmarinus officinalis*)
- Sage (*Salvia officinalis*)
- Summer savory (*Satureja hortensis*)
- Thyme (*Thymus* spp)
- Winter savory (*Satureja montana*)

> **CAUTION** Spices should never be ingested in large quantities, or taken as medicines without medical or professional healthcare advice – turmeric can interact with some pharmaceutical drugs, and nutmeg is dangerous in high doses.

A HERBAL SEASONING

Make this seasoning with home grown herbs in early summer when they are plentiful.

Ingredients

Dried lovage (*Levisticum officinale*)
Marjoram (*Origanum* spp)
Summer or winter savory (*Satureja hortensis* or *S.montana*)
Parsley (*Petroselinum crispum*)
Bay leaves (*Laurus nobilis*)
Sage (*Salvia officinalis*)
Thyme (*Thymus vulgaris*)
Rosemary (*Rosmarinus officinalis*)

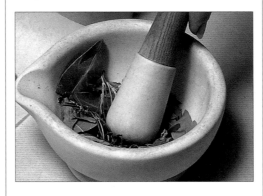

1 Pound equal quantities of dried lovage, marjoram, summer or winter savory and parsley, with half quantities of bay leaf, sage, thyme and rosemary with a mortar and pestle. Pour into airtight jars to store.

Below *Store dried herbs in dark containers.*

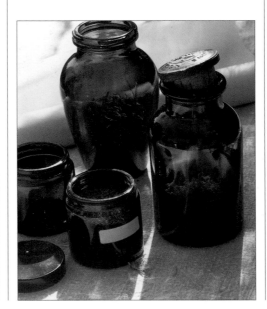

A HOT AND SPICY SEASONING

All these spices stimulate the appetite as well as acting as digestives. Cayenne and ginger help to boost circulation, and cayenne is antibacterial. Add cumin as an optional extra.

Ingredients

Ground mace (*Myristica fragrans*)
Ground coriander (*Coriandrum sativum*)
Ground ginger (*Zingiber officinale*)
Cayenne pepper
Nutmeg (*Myristica fragrans*)

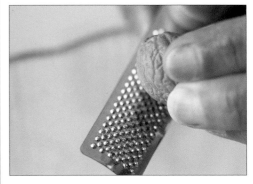

1 Mix together equal quantities of mace, coriander and ginger with one-third as much cayenne pepper and freshly grated nutmeg.

2 Store the mixture in a dark glass jar.

Below *Spices have beneficial properties as well as adding flavour to food.*

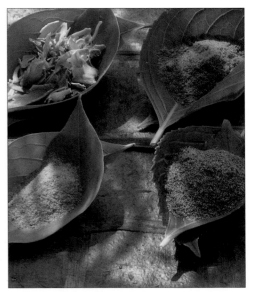

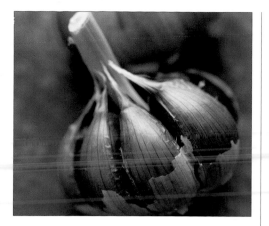

Above *Garlic is good for the circulation.*

Health benefits of garlic

Nature's antibiotic, garlic (*Allium sativum*) has powerful antibacterial and anti-inflammatory properties, and helps the respiratory and other bodily systems to fight infections. It works on the digestive system by supporting beneficial bacteria in the gut, stimulating the secretion of digestive enzymes and aiding absorption of nutrients. It also boosts the circulation and has an effect on lowering blood pressure and cholesterol levels.

For maximum benefit, it should be eaten raw, but it is also efficacious when cooked.

As garlic has a blood-thinning action, it should not be eaten in large quantities if taking anticoagulant medication, or taken as a medicinal extract without medical advice.

Nutritional properties of some herbs	
Herb	**Constituents**
• Chicory	Potassium, folic acid
• Dandelion	Vitamin A
• Garlic	Potassium, vitamins A, B, C
• Kelp	Calcium, iron, iodine, vitamins B_1, B_2, B_{12}
• Nettle	Calcium, iron, vitamins A, C
• Parsley	Calcium, copper, iron, potassium, vitamins A, C
• Watercress	Calcium, folic acid, vitamins A, B_2, C
Fruit	
• Elderberry	Vitamins A, C
• Raspberry	Calcium, vitamin C

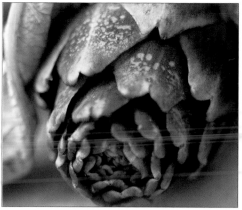

Above *Globe artichoke benefits the liver.*

Health benefits of other foods

• **Globe artichoke** (*Cynara scolymus*) flower heads stimulate the appetite, detoxify the liver and act as a digestive. (The leaves are used in medicinal preparations, but they can be harmful if suffering from gallstones or liver disease and should only be taken on medical advice.)

• **Shiitake mushrooms** are a traditional Japanese remedy, taken in the form of an extract as a restorative tonic and anti-tumour agent. The mushrooms make a useful addition to the diet, helping to boost the immune system.

• **Alfalfa sprouting seeds** contain vitamins C, E, K and beta-carotene. They make an excellent food supplement and can be added to salads or stir-fries.

Below *Seeds, ground and sprinkled on salads, breakfast cereals and cooked dishes, bring health benefits.*

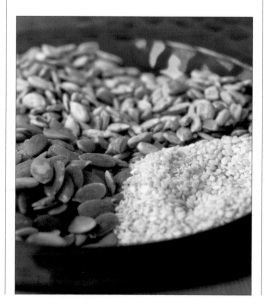

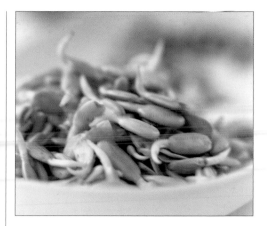

Above *Sprouting seeds are full of vitamins. Add a range of seeds to your cooking whenever possible for their health-boosting attributes.*

• **Safflower oil, olive oil, nuts and avocados** are all good sources of vitamin E, and help to support the immune system.
• **Cloves, nutmeg, cayenne pepper and turmeric** all have antibacterial properties.
• **Cinnamon** helps stabilize blood sugar levels.
• **Caraway, fennel, cardamom and dill** aid digestion.
• **Pumpkin seeds** contain zinc and other trace elements.
• **Sunflower seeds** are rich in B vitamins.

Below *Cinnamon is warming and has been shown to have health benefits particularly for diabetics. Enjoy it in curries, tea and sweet cakes. Even when spices are added sparingly to food, they do more than just provide flavour.*

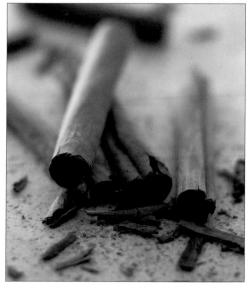

Depression and Feeling Low

Just as with anxiety, depression may have a variety of causes and symptoms. It can be a very serious illness, and for a continued state of depression at any level professional advice should always be sought. But many people have periods of "feeling low", which is a different matter, and at such times herbal teas and tinctures can provide a welcome boost for the spirits.

Symptoms of depression

Depression affects people in different ways and varying degrees. Common symptoms include:

• Low mood.
• Feeling listless.
• Losing interest in everyday pleasures.
• Loss of appetite or overeating.
• Constant tiredess.
• Insomnia or oversleeping.
• Feeling irritable.
• Feeling helpless.

Herbal teas

Teas provide a gentle way to benefit from the properties of herbs, especially if the depression is mild and transient.

• Borage *(Borago officinalis)* flower tea is traditionally associated with courage and strengthening the system. Borage can lift the spirits at stressful times.

To make one cup infuse 10g/⅓ oz fresh borage flowers and 2.5ml/½ tsp dried

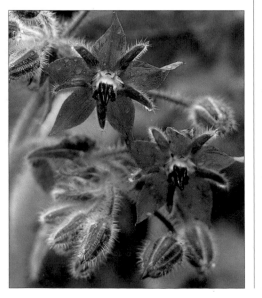

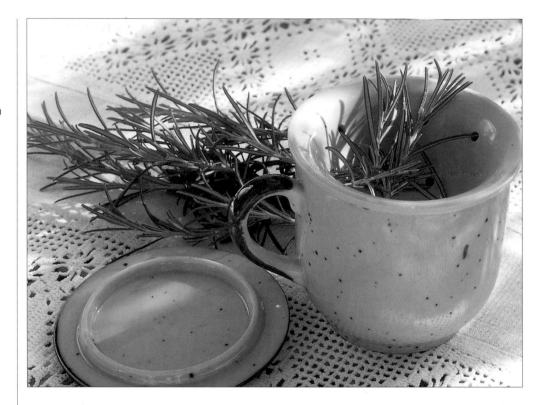

Above A tea infuser is convenient for making a single cup of tea. Rosemary is uplifting.

passion flower in 250ml/8fl oz/1 cup boiling water. Sweeten to taste and drink three times a day.

• To make a **restorative tea** try this powerful combination of herbs. Mix equal parts of dried vervain (*Verbena officinalis*), dried wood betony (*Stachys betonica*), dried mugwort (*Artemisia vulgaris*) and dried rosemary (*Rosmarinus officinalis*). Put 10ml/2 tsp of the mixture into a teapot and fill with boiling water. Allow to steep for 10 minutes and then strain off and discard the dried herbs. Sweeten if preferred with a little honey, and drink one cup of this tea three times a day, but for not more than one week at a time and occasional use only.

CAUTION Wood betony and mugwort are both uterine stimulants and should be avoided during pregnancy and breastfeeding.

Left Borage flowers make a soothing tea for any time of day.

Tincture

A tincture of wild oats (*Avena sativa*), taken in a standard dose, three times a day, is a traditional treatment for mild depression.

Essential oil

Add 6–8 drops essential oil of rose (relaxing) or rosemary (uplifting) to the bath. Or blend 1 drop each essential oil of marjoram, lavender and sandalwood with 5ml/1 tsp almond oil and use as a bath oil.

A healthy diet

Depression illustrates well the connection between body and mind: physical and emotional energy are both depleted when you are in a depressed state. Both will benefit from a healthy diet with plenty of raw, vital foods, nuts, seeds and B vitamins. A multivitamin and mineral supplement may be useful until you feel energetic enough to prepare good food. Try also to cut down on stimulants, such as caffeine, which tend to exhaust both body and mind.

Poor Memory and Concentration

Both memory and concentration can be affected by stress, tiredness and general ill-health. Short-term memory loss is also associated with the ageing process.

Symptoms of poor memory

Losing the memory can be a worrying experience for many people as:
- Levels of alertness may drop.
- Attention span and focus may lessen.
- Memory function may become poor.

Making time for relaxation, taking exercise and eating a nutritious diet will all help to minimize the problem, and herbal treatments can help to make you feel more invigorated and alert. Ginseng (*Panax ginseng*) and ginkgo (*Ginkgo biloba*) are two powerful herbs with a long tradition of use

CAUTION Ginseng and ginkgo are associated with various possible side effects and contra-indications, and they can interact with prescription medicines. For example, ginseng should not be taken by anyone who is suffering from high blood pressure or diabetes, and ginkgo must not be taken while on anticoagulant medication (such as aspirin and warfarin). Only take these remedies under strict medical supervision.

Below *Ginkgo biloba is a powerful herb with mind-enhancing properties.*

in China and the Far East for enhancing mental performance. Modern research studies have confirmed their reputation for strengthening the memory, particularly in the case of ginkgo. Both ginkgo and ginseng are available as ready-made remedies to take on the advice of a qualified practitioner.

Gotu kola (*Centella asiatica*) has been used in India since ancient times for strengthening memory and concentration. It is available in the form of a tincture or tablets, but should only be taken on the advice of a qualified herbal practitioner.

Herbal teas

Favourite teas for improving concentration and general alertness are lemon verbena and rosemary. Use the fresh herb for better taste.
- **Lemon verbena tea** is made using the fresh or dried leaves of the plant and makes a pale golden, lemony tea, which will help to wake up your system. The essential oil of this plant is used by the perfume industry for its invigorating scent. Pour 250ml/8fl oz/1 cup boiling water over a few fresh leaves or 5g/⅛oz dried lemon verbena (*Aloysia triphylla*). Leave to infuse before drinking.
- **Rosemary** Add a small fresh sprig or 5ml/1 tsp of the dried herb to 250ml/8fl oz/1 cup boiling water to make a reviving tea.

Below *Ginseng is said to stimulate the nervous system and increase stamina.*

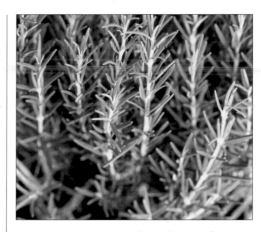

Above *Rosemary contains several active, aromatic oils. Its action is stimulating, as it increases the supply of blood to the brain, keeping the mind clear and aiding concentration. It will also relax nervous tension and combat fatigue.*

Essential oils

Oils to aid concentration include basil, cardamom, peppermint, rosemary, lemon, lemon grass, eucalyptus and cedarwood. Use them singly or in blends of two to three essential oils at a time in a base oil. Use the oil to dab on to a handkerchief or to rub into the pulse points on the wrist, and at the temples.

Below *Essential oils can be vaporized on an essential oil burner, or sprinkled on a handkerchief and the fragrance inhaled.*

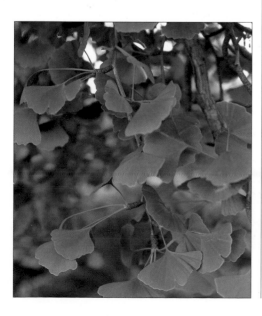

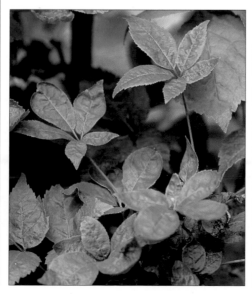

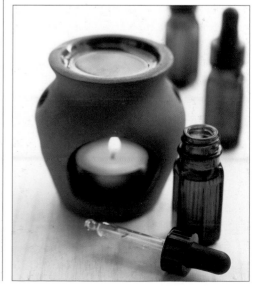

Tiredness and Low Energy

A hectic pace of life, overwork, prolonged stress, illness and even the ageing process can all lead to a constant feeling of tiredness and lack of energy. A healthy diet, high in vitamins (especially A, C, E and B complex), minerals (iron, calcium, magnesium and zinc) and low in refined carbohydrates and sugars, will help boost energy. Alcohol and caffeine drinks are also best avoided and replaced with herb teas and fruit juices.

Causes of tiredness and low energy
Constant feelings of fatigue should make us reassess our lifestyles:
• Eating the wrong foods and drinking too much alcohol can deplete our energy levels.
• A cycle of working too many hours with inadequate time for rest and recuperation can leave us tired or with anxiety, which drains energy.
• Not taking enough exercise makes us feel sluggish. Exercise raises energy levels.

Herbal tea
The gentle action of a herbal infusion provides an uplifting way to start the day. In the early morning, the fresh or dried leaves of lemon verbena (*Aloysia triphylla*) make a cheering drink with a lively flavour to wake up the system. Peppermint also has a gently stimulating effect when taken first thing in the morning.

Revitalizing juice
If you have a juicer, make fresh fruit juices to revitalize the system; they are a good way to increase vitamin content in the diet.

KIWI AND STEM GINGER SPRITZER
A single kiwi fruit contains more than one day's vitamin C requirement. Ginger is a circulatory stimulant that will give your body a much needed boost.

Ingredients
Makes 1 tall glass
2 kiwi fruit
1 piece preserved stem ginger, plus 15ml/
   1 tbsp syrup from the ginger jar
sparkling mineral water

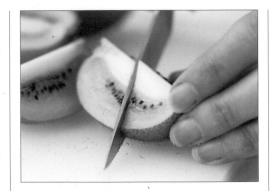

1 Using a sharp knife, roughly chop the kiwi fruit and the ginger.

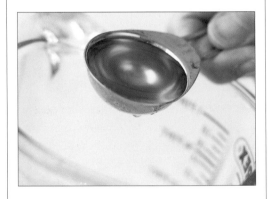

2 Push the ginger and kiwi fruit through a juicer and pour the juice into a jug (pitcher). Stir in the ginger syrup.

3 Pour the juice into a glass, then top up with sparkling mineral water.

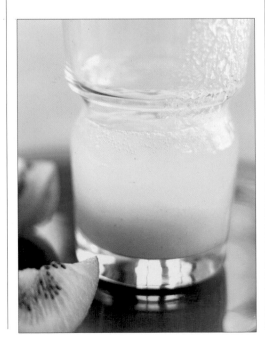

Essential oils
Basil, black pepper, cardamom, pennyroyal, peppermint, pine and rosemary essential oils are re-energizing when used in an oil burner. Use them singly, or experiment with combinations of two or three together, using 8–10 drops in all.

Bath oil
To make an invigorating bath oil, blend
   3 drops essential oil of rosemary and
   2 drops essential oil of camphor with
   5 drops essential oil of peppermint.
Add this blend to 30ml/2 tbsp almond oil. Keep in a stoppered bottle and add 8–10 drops to the water when running a bath.

Bath bag
For a revitalizing mix put equal quantities of dried rosemary (*Rosmarinus officinalis*), peppermint (*Mentha* x *piperita*), lemon thyme (*Thymus* x *citriodorus*) and pine needles into a bath bag to hang over the taps.

Below *A small bag of herbs mixed with essential oils will revive flagging spirits. For a sachet to hang in the car, this pot-pourri mix will help to maintain a clear head. Stir 4 drops each camphor and lemon essential oils into 30ml/2 tbsp ground orris root, then add 25g/1oz each dried lemon verbena (*Aloysia triphylla*), mint, rosemary and thyme and 25g/1oz dried orange and lemon peel. Mix the ingredients together well. Use to fill small sachets. Refresh from time to time with a few drops of essential oil.*

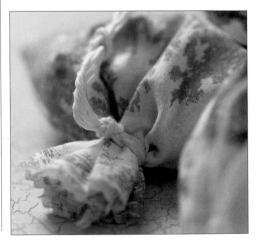

Sleep Disturbances

It is important to distinguish between habitual sleeplessness and a temporary problem, which may be due to some specific worry or anxiety. It would also be sensible not to become obsessed with trying to get a certain amount of sleep, as not everyone needs a full eight hours. But if you are going through a phase of restless nights, there are many ways in which herbs can help. For chronic insomnia seek medical advice.

Causes of sleep disturbances

Many medical conditions can produce sleep disturbances, so too can:
• Anxiety.
• Pain and discomfort.
• External noise.

Herbal teas

An infusion of one or more of these relaxing herbs can help to restore a natural sleep pattern if it has been disturbed by temporary stress and anxiety.
• **Chamomile** (*Chamaemelum nobile* or *Matricaria recutita*) is calming to the nervous system as well as a digestive, and is one of the best bedtime drinks for those who have difficulty dropping off. If the tea is made with dried chamomile flowers (rather than a ready-made teabag), it can be combined with an equal quantity of sweet marjoram (*Origanum majorana*).
• **Lime blossom** (*Tilia europaea*) and **elderflower** (*Sambucus nigra*) make a pleasant-tasting tea that is gently soporific. For maximum effect, add a dash of nutmeg and sweeten with honey.
• **Passion flower** (*Passiflora incarnata*) is known for its sedative properties, and for relieving nervous conditions such as palpitations. It makes a relaxing tea. You can also mix it with an equal quantity of other sedative herbs, including wood betony (*Stachys officinalis*), vervain (*Verbena officinalis*) and mugwort (*Artemisia vulgaris*).
• Put 5ml/1 tsp each dried passion flower (*Passiflora incarnata*), vervain (*Verbena officinalis*) and wood betony into a pot and pour in 600ml/1 pint/2½ cups boiling water water. Leave to infuse for 5 minutes. Strain.

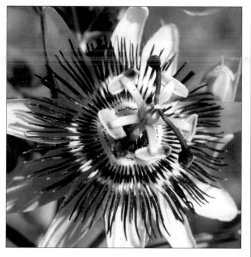

Above *Passion flower is easy to grow. The flowers have gently sedative properties.*

CAUTION Wood betony and mugwort are uterine stimulants, and should not be used during pregnancy or while breastfeeding.

Drink 1–2 cups of this gently sedative mixture daily, for not more than 2 weeks.

Tincture

A tincture made with the flowers of sweet violet (*Viola odorata*) taken in a standard dose, helps induce restfulness.

Essential oils

Chamomile, juniper, lavender, marjoram, neroli, sandalwood and lemon essential oils can be used in an oil burner, singly or in combinations of two or three together.
• For a massage oil to help you sleep, add 4 drops each of chamomile, lemon and sandalwood to 30ml/2 tbsp base oil.
• A simple way to promote restful sleep is to sprinkle a few drops of essential oil of lavender on to your pillow or handkerchief.
• A small cushion filled with sleep-inducing hops and lavender, placed behind your head, or under your main pillow, is a gentle way to encourage a restful night.
• Adding a few drops of lavender oil to a warm, not hot, bath taken just before going to bed will also have a calming effect on the body.

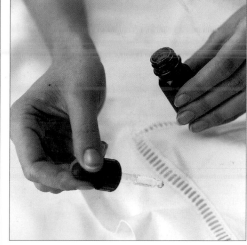

Above *A few drops of essential oil of lavender on the pillow should ensure a restful night.*

SLEEP TIME OIL SPRAY

Spray the room before you go to sleep with this relaxing fragrance. You can also use it at any time to provide a calming atmosphere. Once mixed, keep the oils in a cool dark place away from a source of heat.

Ingredients

25ml/5 tsp grapeseed oil
25ml/5 tsp almond oil
25ml/5 tsp jojoba oil
10ml/2 tsp rosewater
10ml/2 tsp glycerine
20 drops each lavender and chamomile essential oils

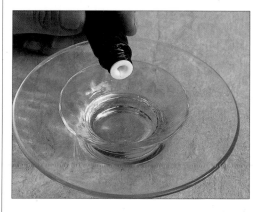

Mix the first five ingredients together, then stir in the essential oils, mixing well. Transfer to a clean 100ml/3½fl oz spray bottle. Shake before use.

Headaches

Ranging in severity from mild and bearable to severe and debilitating, headaches can be very disruptive to life. Herbs may be helpful in relieving headaches that are brought on by anxiety or tension. Fresh or dried herbs can be made into teas; or a lavender infusion can be used for a compress.

Causes of headaches

Headaches can develop for a number of reasons; usually they are related to some obvious cause such as:

• Nasal congestion or sinusitis.

• Eye strain, fatigue or tension.

• Stress or worries, with muscle spasms in the neck leading to head pains.

• Poor posture – many jobs create special problems: for instance, computer operators often suffer from eye strain and stiff, aching shoulders or neck muscles, and consequently headaches.

Herbal teas

At the earliest signs of a headache, taking a tea made from one of the following herbs can stop it in its tracks.

• **Chamomile** (*Matricaria recutita*) is good for bilious headaches stemming from over-eating, or indigestion, where there is a dull, throbbing pain on top of the head.

• **Lime blossom** (*Tilia europaea*) soothes the nerves and is very helpful for tension headaches; it can be mixed with peppermint for a more uplifting effect.

• **Peppermint** (*Mentha piperita*) works well for digestive or sinus headaches, especially where the head feels hot.

• **Rosemary** (*Rosmarinus officinalis*) is good for headaches related to exhaustion or depression, and also for bilious heavy heads.

• **Hangover remedy** Put 5ml/1 tsp dried vervain (*Verbena officinalis*) and 2.5ml/½ tsp lavender (*Lavandula*) flowers in a teapot and pour over 600ml/1 pint/2½ cups boiling water. Allow to steep for 10 minutes, then strain. Sweeten with a little honey, if you like. Sip this tea as often as you like throughout the day until you start to feel better, but remember that prevention is better than cure!

Severe headaches

Persistent headaches can be debilitating and if they become a recurrent problem, you should get medical advice. Conditions such as very high blood pressure, meningitis or even brain tumours are relatively rare causes of headaches, but they need professional treatment. Severe, unexplained or persistent headaches should be checked out carefully by a medical practitioner, but most headaches and their causes can be identified and cured at home. Where some kind of accident has resulted in, say, a whiplash injury, professional help is required, and you could consult a manipulative therapist such as a chiropractor or an osteopath for treatment.

Compress

Headaches are often caused by tension in the neck and upper back muscles. This can prevent adequate blood supply to the head and thus lead to pain. Both massage and exercise can be a great help in easing this kind of headache. A cool compress may also help. An infusion of a cooling herb such as mint can be used to make a compress. Lavender is also popular, but if you find the fragrance too strong, leave out the essential oil content in the recipe below.

LAVENDER COMPRESS FOR A HEADACHE

Place a cool lavender compress across the forehead to relieve a tension headache. Sit and relax with the compress in place. As soon as the compress gets warm, soak it again in the infusion and reapply.

Ingredients

25g/1oz dried lavender (*Lavandula* spp)
600ml/1 pint/2½ cups boiling water
3–4 drops lavender essential oil
10ml/2 tsp lavender tincture

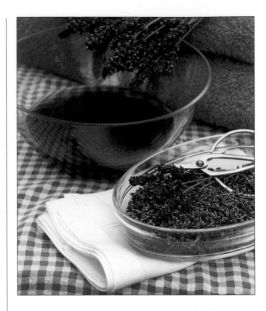

1 Put the dried lavender in a bowl and pour the boiling water over it. Leave to stand for 1 hour, then strain. When cool, mix in the essential oil and tincture.

2 Fold a piece of soft cotton fabric into a loose pad. Soak it in the lavender infusion and wring it out lightly.

Below *Holding a pad to your head with a few drops each of sweet marjoram and lemon balm essential oils can relieve a tension headache. If the headache persists, try adding a few drops of chamomile* (Chamaemelum nobile). *While using a compress it is better to try and relax than to continue with your usual daily activities.*

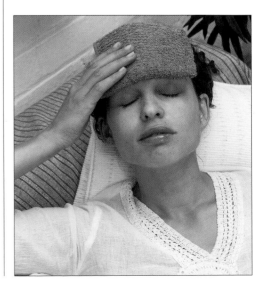

Migraine

Anyone who has experienced migraine will know that it is more than a severe headache. Diet may be a key factor. Tea, coffee, alcohol (especially red wine), cheese, chocolate, tomatoes and eggs have all been implicated as triggers. Massaging the neck, in between attacks, may help, and herbal teas are soothing and comforting.

Symptoms of migraine
- Intense and uncomfortable headache.
- Acute pains, often over one eye.
- Disturbed vision or flashing lights.
- Nausea or vomiting.
- Sensitivity to bright light.

Herbal teas
Taking a herbal tea in the early stages may help reduce the effects of a migraine. You could also try drinking one of these infusions regularly in place of tea or coffee.
- **Chamomile** (*Matricaria recutita*) for dull, throbbing headache with a feeling of queasiness – add a little ginger (*Zingiber officinalis*) to relieve more severe nausea.
- **Rosemary** (*Rosmarinus officinalis*) is good where stress is a trigger for migraines, and where local warmth gives relief.
- For a **soothing tea** drink 1 cup of this herbal tea a day for up to one week. Put 5ml/1 tsp dried wood betony and

Below *Feverfew is an age-old migraine cure.*

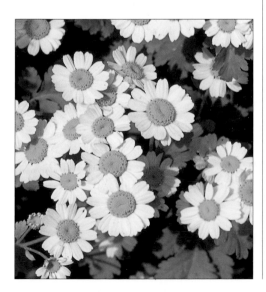

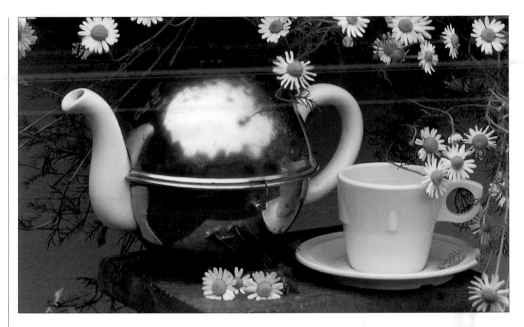

Above *Chamomile tea makes a soothing drink at any time of day for those prone to migraine.*

2.5ml/½ tsp dried lavender (*Lavandula*) or rosemary (*Rosmarinus officinalis*) in a cup. Top up with boiling water and steep for 10 minutes, then strain.

Feverfew
This is one of the herbal remedies of which most people have heard, as it was hailed as a "wonder cure" for migraine in the 1970s after a Welsh doctor's wife found that it put a stop to her chronic migraine attacks. Since then the use of feverfew (*Tanacetum parthenium*) has undergone much scientific research, which has largely confirmed its effectiveness but also revealed its side effects and risks. It should be used with caution.

CAUTION It was once considered safe to eat one or two fresh small leaves of feverfew a day, with food, as a preventive measure, but it has now been established that feverfew is potentially toxic and can cause allergic reactions, mouth ulcers and stomach upsets. It also interacts with prescription blood-thinning medication, such as aspirin and warfarin, and should not be taken without medical advice and supervision.

Compress
A cool compress placed across the forehead may be helpful. It is probably best to use plain water for this, as the sense of smell is often heightened or altered during a migraine, and any strongly scented herb is likely to make matters worse. You could try adding a few fresh mint leaves to the water for the compress, for a hint of fragrance.

Treating migraine

A migraine can be triggered by hormone changes, stress, stuffy atmospheres, noises, smells and certain foods. Repeated attacks call for professional help: self-help treatments are largely for preventive use.

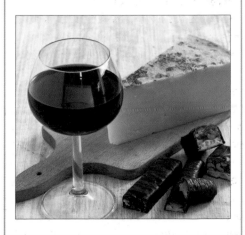

Colds and Influenza

Once a cold has developed it generally has to run its course, but herbal treatments can help to relieve symptoms and also stop the cold leading on to persistent catarrh or a deeper infection. Influenza is a much more serious complaint than a bad cold, as anyone who has suffered it will know, but some of its symptoms may also be eased by preparations appropriate for colds.

Symptoms of colds and flu

Everyone is familiar with the symptoms of a cold. At their worst, colds can leave us feeling low and uninterested in life and with:
- Sore throats
- Coughs
- Headaches
- Blocked sinuses or runny nose.

Herbal teas

One of the herbalists' most traditional standbys for colds is still one of the best: make an infusion of equal amounts of peppermint (*Mentha x piperita*), elderflower (*Sambucus nigra*) and yarrow (*Achillea millefolium*). Taken hot just before going to bed, it will induce a sweat. You could also add a pinch of **cayenne powder**, a favourite North American Indian remedy: it stimulates the circulation.
- **Ginger** (*Zingiber officinalis*) – use a ginger herbal tea bag or make an infusion from grated fresh root ginger.

Below *Ginger tea is warming and ideal for relieving the symptoms of colds.*

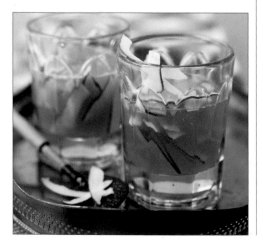

GARLIC COLD SYRUP

The health-giving properties of garlic have been recognized since ancient Egyptian times, when it was thought to bestow strength. Modern research confirms that garlic has antibacterial properties.

It is also antiviral, a decongestant and may help the body combat infection. Combine it with honey, which is soothing and mildly antiseptic, in a syrup to prevent or relieve the symptoms of colds and flu. Take 10–15ml/2–3 tsp three times a day.

Ingredients

1 head of garlic (*Allium sativum*)
300ml/½ pint/1¼ cups water
juice of ½ lemon
30ml/2 tbsp honey

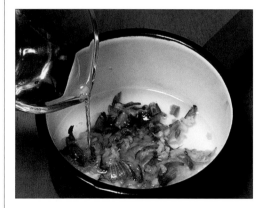

1 Crush the garlic cloves – there is no need to peel them – and put them in a pan with the water. Bring to the boil and simmer gently for 20 minutes. Cover the pan to prevent the liquid evaporating.

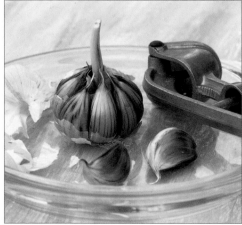

TIP Make the most of garlic's beneficial properties by adding it to food on a daily basis. You could also consider taking it in capsule form.

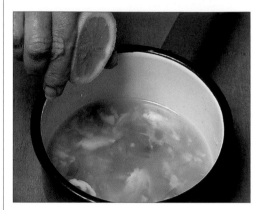

2 Add the lemon juice and honey and simmer for a further 2–3 minutes. Allow the mixture to cool slightly, then strain it into a clean, dark glass jar or bottle with an airtight lid. Keep for 2–3 weeks in the refrigerator.

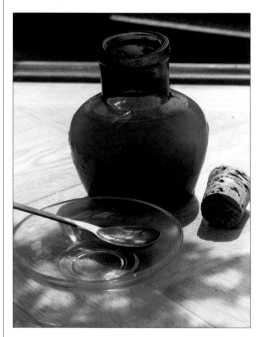

Above *Garlic syrup, made with honey and lemon, makes an excellent cold cure.*

Left *Look for plump fresh cloves when buying garlic. Its beneficial properties are most potent when it is eaten raw, but when cooked it still has some potency.*

CAMPHOR AND EUCALYPTUS VAPOUR RUB

This ointment contains decongestant oils to relieve blocked nasal cavities. It should be rubbed on to the throat or chest or used as an inhalant.

Ingredients
50g/2oz petroleum jelly
15g/1 tbsp dried lavender (*Lavandula* spp)
6 drops eucalyptus essential oil
4 drops camphor essential oil

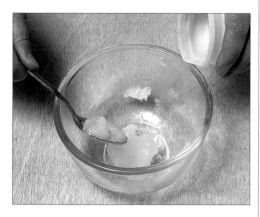

1 Melt the petroleum jelly in a bowl over a pan of simmering water, stir in the lavender and heat gently for 30 minutes.

2 Strain the liquid jelly through muslin, leave to cool slightly, then add the essential oils. Pour into a clean jar and leave until set. This will keep for 6 months.

3 Rub on to the chest or melt 15ml/1 tbsp in a bowl of hot water and inhale the steam.

Essential oils

The warmth and steam of a scented bath at bedtime will clear a stuffy head and help you sleep. Add 3–4 drops each of eucalyptus, thyme and lavender essential oils.

• Alternatively fill a bath bag with lavender (*Lavandula* spp), thyme and a 2.5cm/ 1in piece of fresh ginger (*Zingiber officinale*), grated, and hang it under the running tap to scent the bath water.

• Vaporizing essential oils in a burner will help with breathing difficulties when you are suffering from a cold. Try one of the following combinations: 3 drops each eucalyptus, tea tree and lavender, or 4 drops eucalyptus, 2 drops hyssop and 2 drops thyme.

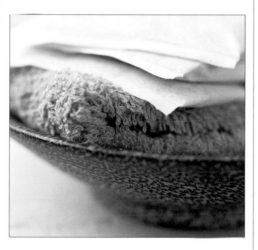

Above *A bath bag filled with head-clearing herbs relieves a stuffy nose. Make your own small cotton bag and add your choice of fresh or dried herbs.*

MUSTARD FOOT BATH

This has long been a popular treatment for colds and chills. It has a warming effect and is extremely comforting.

Ingredients
15g/1 tbsp mustard powder
2.2 litres/4 pints/9 cups hot water

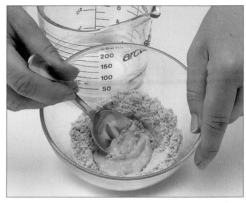

1 Stir the mustard and a small quantity of water together in a small bowl, stirring until the mustard dissolves.

2 Put the remaining hot water in the foot bath and add the dissolved mustard. Stir well.

3 Immerse the feet while the water is still hot. Re-heat the water if required.

Below *A mustard foot bath is a traditional treatment for colds. You could also try adding stimulating herbs such as rosemary (*Rosmarinus officinalis*) to the water.*

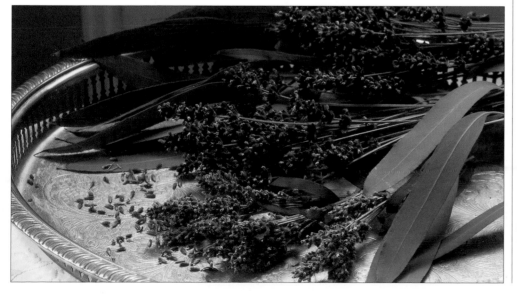

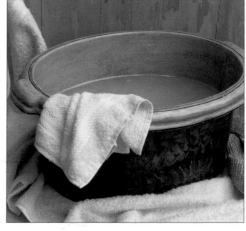

Left *Lavender and eucalyptus have a decongestant action.*

Coughs

A cough is a natural reflex reaction to any irritation, inflammation or blockage in the airways and is nature's way of keeping the bronchial tubes open and clear. It often accompanies an infection such as a cold but may also be due to breathing in dust or some other pollutant or allergen and will be self-limiting.

Causes of coughs

• Coughs often accompany colds, when we are run down and feeling low.
• Coughs can be a response to a much more serious underlying medical issue such as asthma, bronchitis or cancer.

> **CAUTION** The herbal treatments recommended here are for the type of cough associated with common colds. Self-treatment is not appropriate for more serious or persistent coughs, or for one that accompanies a chest infection such as bronchitis. Always seek medical advice under these circumstances.

Herbal teas

A herbal infusion can be very soothing for troublesome, tickly coughs.
• **Coltsfoot** (*Tussilago farfara*) is a traditional herb for a cough, particularly for one that is irritating and spasmodic, and is recommended by many herbalists. It has a soothing effect, loosens mucus and reduces the spasm of a cough. Use the dried leaf of coltsfoot to make an infusion or buy as a standardized extract. Not to be taken during pregnancy or while breastfeeding.
• **Hyssop** (*Hyssopus officinalis*) is calming and relaxing and a gentle expectorant. Use the fresh or dried leaf, or the flower heads, to make a tea. As hyssop tastes quite bitter, honey and a little freshly squeezed orange juice (which also adds valuable vitamin C) will make it more palatable.
• **Marshmallow** (*Althaea officinalis*) is a herb whose demulcent properties make it highly soothing to inflamed bronchial tubes. It is especially useful for a harsh, dry cough to ease the soreness. It is best taken as an infusion, made from the fresh or dried flowers, or as a decoction of the dried roots.
• **Thyme** (*Thymus vulgaris*) is well known for its antiseptic properties; an infusion of fresh or dried thyme helps relieve a dry cough linked with a respiratory infection. Lemon thyme (*T. citriodorus*) can also be used.
• **White horehound** (*Marrubium vulgare*), used as an expectorant, helps free up thick, sticky mucus when you have a chesty cold. Make a tea with the fresh or dried herb. Sweeten with honey to taste and add a dash of lemon juice for a burst of vitamin C.
• **Chamomile** (*Chamaemelum nobile*), **elderflower** (*Sambucus nigra*) and **peppermint** (*Mentha* x *piperita*) make a palatable, soothing tea that will help to ease a troublesome cough. Put 2.5g/½ tsp each of dried peppermint, elderflower and chamomile in a small teapot. Add a pinch each dried lavender and ginger and pour over 250ml/8fl oz/1 cup boiling water. Infuse for 2–3 minutes, then strain into a cup. Stir in 5ml/1 tsp honey. Add a slice of lemon.

Below *If you are susceptible to coughs, make up a batch of linctus at the onset of winter. Drink plenty of herb teas to keep the throat moist. This will also help relieve the discomfort of a sore throat.*

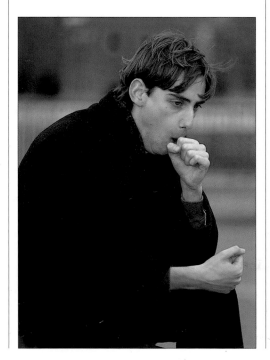

THYME AND BORAGE COUGH LINCTUS

Borage and thyme combine well to make a pleasant-tasting linctus.

Ingredients
25g/1oz fresh or 15g/½ oz dried thyme (*Thymus* spp)
25g/1oz fresh or 15g/½ oz dried borage (*Borago officinale*)
2 x 5cm/2in cinnamon sticks
600ml/1 pint/2½ cups water
juice of 1 small lemon
100g/4oz/½ cup honey

1 Put the herbs into a pan with the cinnamon and water. Bring to the boil, cover and simmer for 20 minutes.

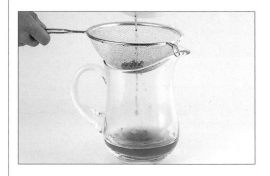

2 Strain off the herbs. Return the liquid to the pan. Simmer, uncovered, until reduced by half. Add the lemon juice and honey and simmer for 5 mintues. Bottle and store for up to 2 months. Take 5ml/1 tsp, as required.

Below *The antiseptic properties of thyme make it ideal for treating coughs.*

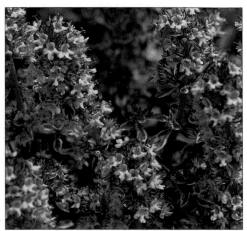

Sore Throats

With increased airborne pollution and the dry atmosphere in air conditioned offices, sore throats are becoming more common throughout the year, and not just in the winter months. The irritation can range from an annoying tickle to a rasping soreness that makes speech difficult. Gargling with a strong herbal infusion or sipping a warming decoction will help ease the discomfort.

CAUTION A sore throat may be linked to another infection or be a symptom of a serious health problem, and if it persists for more than a week, seek medical advice.

HYSSOP AND HOREHOUND GARGLE

Both hyssop (*Hyssopus officinalis*) and white horehound (*Marrubium vulgare*) have been considered by herbalists to be effective remedies for sore throats. They also combine well to make a strong gargle. Make an infusion of the leaves and flowering tops of both herbs, following the directions given here for thyme and sage gargle. Sipping herb teas can also bring relief for a sore throat. Choose from any you find palatable.

Below *Lemon offers vitamin C, which can be taken in drinks to soothe a sore throat.*

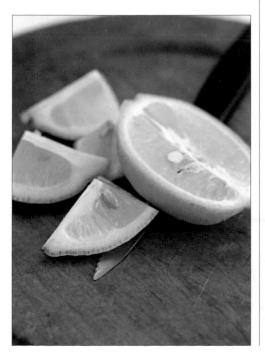

THYME AND SAGE GARGLE

Gargling with a strong herbal infusion or sipping a warming decoction will help ease the discomfort of a sore throat. When fresh herbs are not available, dried ones can be substituted, using 30ml/2 tbsp in 600ml/ 1 pint/2½ cups water.

Gargle with this mixture at the first sign of a sore throat. It can also be taken internally, 10ml/2 tsp at a time, 2–3 times a day. Use within 2 days.

Ingredients
small handful each fresh sage (*Salvia officinalis*) and thyme (*Thymus* spp) leaves, roughly chopped
600ml/1 pint/2½ cups boiling water
30ml/2 tbsp cider vinegar
10ml/2 tsp honey
5ml/1 tsp cayenne pepper

Put the chopped leaves into a pot, pour in the boiling water, cover and leave to steep for 30 minutes. Strain off the liquid and stir in the cider vinegar, honey and cayenne.

Below: *Hyssop* (Hyssopus officinalis) *(with blue flowers) and horehound* (Marrubium vulgare) *(far right) combine well in a gargle for sore throats.*

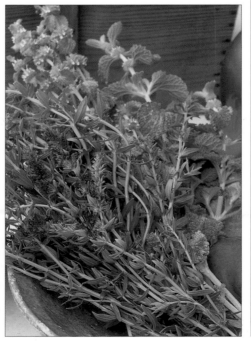

GINGER AND LEMON DECOCTION

Lemon provides vitamin C, while ginger is warming and stimulating and encourages sweating to eliminate toxins and dispel mucus and catarrh. This decoction will keep for 2–3 days.

Ingredients
115g/4oz piece of fresh root ginger
600ml/1 pint/2½ cups water
juice and rind of 1 lemon
pinch of cayenne pepper

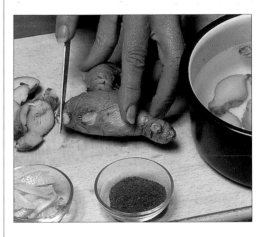

1 Slice the ginger root – there is no need to peel it – and put it in a pan with the water, lemon rind and cayenne. Always use an enamelled rather than an aluminium pan.

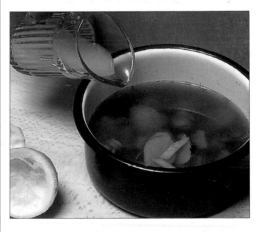

2 Bring to the boil, cover the pan and simmer for 20 minutes. Remove from the heat and add the lemon juice.

3 Drink a small cupful at a time, sweetened with honey.

Indigestion

Indigestion is a general term for the discomfort caused by digestive disturbances. Usually it is a temporary problem brought about by eating too much or the wrong kind of food or from drinking excess alcohol. It can also be stress related. Short-term digestive problems of this kind generally respond quite well to herbal treatment. Longer-term digestive pains may have more serious causes for which medical advice should always be taken.

Symptoms of indigestion
• Abdominal discomfort and flatulence.
• Upset stomach.
• Heartburn.

Herbal teas
Infusions can be very helpful in easing indigestion. Choose from the following.
• **Chamomile** (*Matricaria recutita*) is calming and is good for the effects of over-eating and for stress-related indigestion.
• **Lemon balm** (*Melissa officinalis*) settles a churning stomach and is another good herb for nervous indigestion. Make the tea with the fresh leaf.
• **Peppermint** (*Mentha x piperita*) is good for indigestion accompanied by flatulence and a bloated abdomen.
• **Dill** (*Anethum graveolens*) acts gently to ease indigestion and can even be given to babies and young children. Allow 5ml/1 tsp lightly crushed dill seed to 250ml/8fl oz/ 1 cup of water and boil for 10 minutes. Strain and allow to cool before drinking.
• **Fennel seed** (*Foeniculum vulgare*) is good for flatulence and acid indigestion. See the recipe for fennel seed tea opposite.
• **Marigold** (*Calendula officinalis*) and **lemon verbena** (*Aloysia triphylla*) make a refreshing digestive. This tisane is reputed to be excellent for purifying the blood and aiding digestion. The verbena gives an intense lemon flavour and the marigold adds a peppery note. Mix 50g/2oz dried marigold petals with 25g/1oz dried lemon verbena leaves. Store in an airtight container. Prepare an infusion using 15g/½oz herb to 600ml/1 pint/ 2½ cups boiling water.

GINGER JUICE WITH PINEAPPLE
Fresh root ginger is one of the best natural cures for indigestion. It also helps to settle upset stomachs, whether caused by food poisoning or motion sickness. In this unusual fruity blend, it is mixed with fresh, juicy pineapple and sweet-tasting carrot. It can be juiced up in seconds and tastes delicious. Make one for breakfast for general indigestion. For an upset stomach take weak ginger tea on its own.

Ingredients
Makes 1 glass
½ small pineapple
25g/1oz fresh root ginger
1 carrot
ice cubes

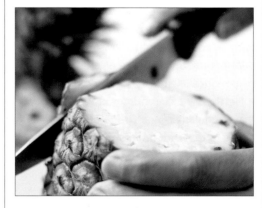

1 Cut away the skin from the pineapple, then halve and remove the core. Roughly slice the pineapple flesh, reserving half for another use.

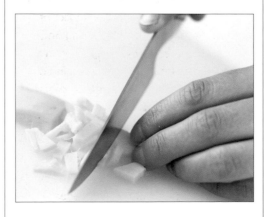

2 Peel and chop the ginger and chop the carrot into large chunks.

TIP Before preparing a pineapple for juicing or cutting it into chunks or rings, cut off the leafy top, turn the pineapple upside down in a dish and leave it for half an hour – this makes it juicier.

The quickest and easiest way to cut up a pineapple is to cut off the top and bottom edges. Then slice the skin away from the sides using a sharp knife. Carefully trim away the eyes, without discarding too much of the fruit.

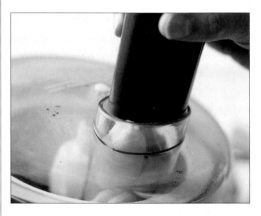

3 Push the carrot, ginger and pineapple through a juicer and pour into a glass. Add ice cubes and serve immediately.

Below *Ginger is a well known cure for many everyday ailments.*

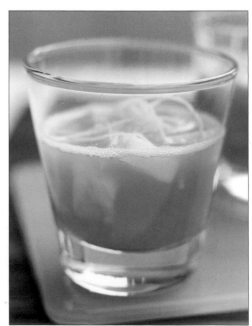

Acidity and Heartburn

Many people get occasional bouts of acid dyspepsia, as this kind of indigestion is known, usually related to a temporary problem such as having eaten rich, spicy foods or having eaten too quickly. If the symptoms happen very regularly, you may need to look more carefully at what you eat and how fast you eat it. If there is persistent discomfort, seek professional treatment. When excess acid leaks back up into the gullet, this inflames and irritates the lining of the oesophagus and the feeling of heartburn is produced. Taking antacid tablets regularly may not only mask underlying problems, but can also be counterproductive as the stomach tries to compensate by creating more acid.

Symptoms of heartburn
• A burning sensation near the breastbone.
• Mild discomfort.

Herbal teas
To relieve a temporary bout of heartburn, choose from the following teas. For repeated symptoms of acidity and heartburn, make the infusions stronger by increasing the quantity of herb used (by half as much again) and leaving to steep for a few minutes longer.
• **Chamomile** (*Matricaria recutita*) is an anti-inflammatory remedy and relaxant that helps the whole digestive tract; if acid symptoms are related to stress and/or over-eating of rich foods, this herb makes an excellent choice.

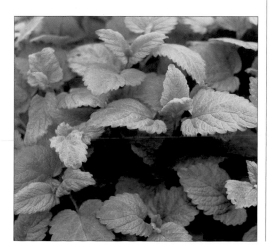

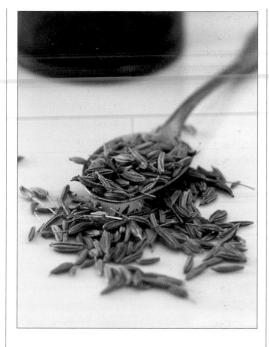

Above *Known for their digestive properties, fennel seeds, along with caraway seeds, are often handed round after meals in eastern countries as aids to digestion. They may be in their natural state or coated in sugar.*

• **Lemon balm** (*Melissa officinalis*) is another excellent herb where the condition is caused by stress; always use the fresh leaves.
• **Meadowsweet** (*Filipendula ulmaria*), although chemically related to aspirin, it is soothing for an inflamed stomach. It may need to be avoided by those who have a hypersensitivity to salicylates such as aspirin. It also reduces acidity.
• **Slippery elm** (*Ulmus fulva*), the powdered bark of a native North American elm tree, is highly soothing to the inflamed gullet or stomach. It may be taken by mixing 5ml/ 1 tsp of the pure powder in a little warm water – it lives up to its name, slipping down easily, coating and soothing the membranes.
• **Fennel seed (*Foeniculum vulgare*) tea** With a mild aniseed flavour, fennel is a diuretic and has a calming effect on the stomach, easing flatulence and indigestion. Caraway seeds can be prepared in the same way, or combined with fennel in equal

Left *Lemon balm makes a soothing tea for reducing stress.*

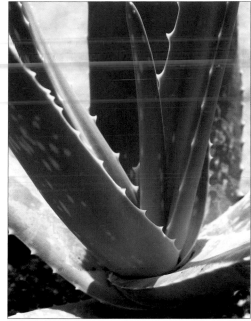

Above *Aloe vera, a traditional digestive remedy, should be used with medical advice.*

quantities. Put 5ml/1 tsp fennel seeds in a small pan with 250ml/8fl oz/1 cup of water and boil for 10 minutes. Strain and allow to cool before drinking. Add a slice of orange or a sliver of orange rind for extra flavour.

Aloe vera juice
The juice of the aloe vera plant has a long history of use as a remedy for digestive problems. While this, and its positive effect on the immune system, have been confirmed by research studies, some species used in medicinal products are potentially toxic. It is therefore essential, if taking aloe vera internally, to do so with professional advice and under medical supervision.

Digestive herbs in food
• **Sage** (*Salvia officinalis*), like many culinary herbs, aids digestion. It has a robust flavour, which stands up to long cooking processes and goes well with cheese and meat dishes.
• **Parsley** (*Petroselinum crispum*) and **chervil** (*Anthriscus cerefolium*) are also helpful to the digestion when used in cooking.
• **Caraway** and **fennel seeds**, well known for their digestive properties, can be added to dishes or chewed after a meal.

Acne

This skin condition is very common during puberty, and may continue into later life for some people. Increasing levels of hormones during adolescence lead to greater activity of the skin's sebaceous glands, and if this becomes too great, excessive amounts of sebum, the skin's natural oily lubricant, are produced. This in turn can cause the glands and hair follicles to become blocked and infected. Diet is an important factor in treating acne, and herbal remedies should be aimed at cleansing the whole system as well as the skin.

The most common reaction of most people who suffer from acne is to squeeze the spots; this almost always serves to spread the infection into the surrounding tissues, and if done repeatedly can damage the local skin areas, producing scarring. Any programme of treatment therefore needs to include a lot of self-help to be successful.

The natural therapies offer the most successful and sensible ways to improve the condition and rebalance the skin. The best approach is to combine local, external cleansing with internal treatment; all therapies are likely to emphasize the importance of diet in treating acne. Where acne persists for years after adolescence,

Below *Milk thistle (*Silybum marianum*) is a detoxifying herb with antioxidant properties that is often recommended for treating acne.*

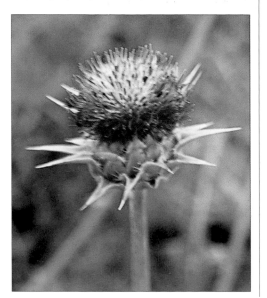

there may be an a hormonal imbalance that needs to be addressed, and again there are natural remedies that may be used – seek professional treatment if necessary.

Herbal teas
Drinking teas made from detoxifying herbs will help to reduce inflammation. Choose from the following and drink three or four cups during the day: red clover (*Trifolium pratense*), nettle (*Urtica dioica*), cleavers (*Galium aparine*) and milk thistle (*Silybum marianum*), singly or in combination.

Infusion
Instead of using soap, which removes the acid mantle of the skin and thus increases the susceptibility to infection, rinse the face with a herbal infusion.

Red clover is an excellent blood and tissue cleanser and has a gentle action: as well as drinking it as a tea, an infusion of red clover can be used externally to carefully bathe inflamed spots.

Decoction
Dandelion root (*Taraxacum officinale*), taken as a decoction, is helpful in improving the detoxifying action of the liver, which can help to clear the skin. It also has a gentle laxative action, taking pressure away from the skin as an organ of elimination.

Tincture
Echinacea (*E. purpurea*) is one of the best all-purpose immune stimulants, aiding resistance to infection. It can be taken in conjunction with the herbal treatments suggested above, to help the detoxification process. It is best taken in the form of a ready-made tincture, following the manufacturer's directions on dosage. Do not take for more than 2–3 weeks at a time and do not resume taking it within a month.

Steam inhalation
Regular steam inhalations with juniper can help clear blocked pores or blackheads. Add 3–4 drops juniper oil or fresh juniper leaves and berries to a basin of water.

HERBAL CLEANSING RINSE
This rinse is best made fresh each day. For early morning use, make it the night before and keep it in a cool place, in a covered container. Elderflower and marigold have soothing, anti-inflammatory properties and lavender is antiseptic in action. Witch hazel is an astringent, to help tone the skin.

Ingredients
15ml/1 tbsp each dried elderflower, lavender and marigold petals
5ml/1 tsp distilled witch hazel
600ml/1 pint/2½ cups boiling water

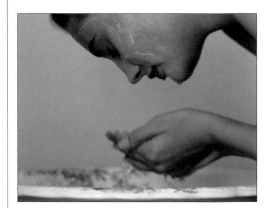

Put the dried herbs into a bowl and pour in the boiling water. Leave for 20 minutes before straining into a larger bowl. Stir in the witch hazel and use to rinse the face.

Below *Dandelion has a detoxifying action.*

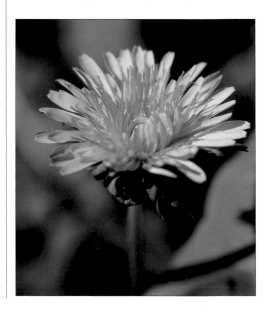

Athlete's Foot

Athlete's foot is a common fungal infection that affects the skin of the foot (not just those of athletes). It is highly contagious and thrives in warm, moist environments, such as swimming pool changing rooms and showers. Symptoms are an itchy, red rash between the toes, which may then blister and become sore. It can also spread to toenails, making them flaky and yellow. Self-treatment with herbal remedies may help to clear it. If it persists it is best to seek professional advice.

It is most important to keep the affected area cool and dry. Pay scrupulous attention to hygiene as the fungus can accumulate under the nails, causing the infection to spread between the toes.

Prevention
• Do not share towels.
• Wear plastic shoes in communal changing areas and around swimming pools.
• Wash feet daily and dry thoroughly between the toes.
• Do not wear shoes without socks or tights.
• Change your socks or tights daily.

Tinctures
• Marigold (*Calendula officinalis*) and myrrh (*Commiphora myrrha*) have antifungal properties and can be applied directly to the skin as tinctures. Buy them as ready-made products, or make your own tinctures following the instructions on page 28.

Internal treatments
To prevent recurrent infection, it may help to take internal remedies to bolster the immune system. Take garlic regularly, either in food, or in capsule form (but not without first seeking professional healthcare advice if you are taking other medication), and perhaps a short course of echinacea tincture (see opposite). Aloe vera juice may be helpful, but should only be taken with professional advice. Drink plenty of herbal teas with antifungal and digestive properties, including thyme (*Thymus* spp), chamomile (*Chamaemelum nobile*), marigold (*Calendula officinalis*) and rose (*Rosa* spp).

ANTIFUNGAL FOOT BATH
Make a strong infusion of marigold (*Calendula officinalis*) and thyme (*Thymus vulgaris*), or ginger and cinnamon, and soak your feet in it twice a day for 15 minutes, taking care to dry them well afterwards and dust with antifungal foot powder. The cider vinegar in this foot bath helps to restore the pH balance of the skin, which becomes over-alkaline when suffering from athlete's foot. Both myrrh and tea tree oil have antifungal properties.

Ingredients
25g/1oz dried sage (*Salvia officinalis*)
25g/1oz dried pot marigold (*Calendula officinalis*) flowers
1 large aloe vera leaf, chopped
15ml/1 tbsp myrrh granules
2¼ pints/9 cups water
10 drops tea tree essential oil
60ml/4 tbsp cider vinegar

1 Simmer the herbs and myrrh in the water for 20 minutes.

2 Leave to cool a little, then strain and add the tea tree oil and the cider vinegar.

Below *Soaking the feet in a decoction of antifungal herbs and oils helps combat this contagious condition and can provide instant relief to itching feet.*

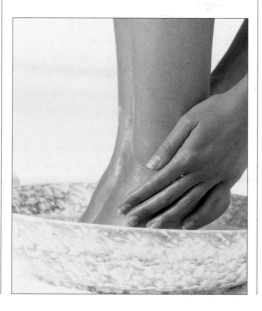

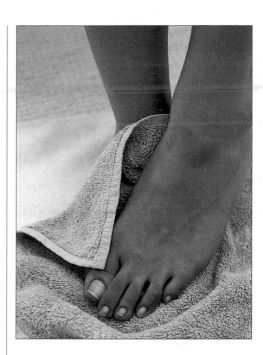

Above *Keeping feet clean and dry helps to prevent athlete's foot.*

MARIGOLD AND MYRRH FOOT POWDER
Talcum powder helps keep feet dry and sweat-free, and a mixture incorporating antifungal ingredients, such as marigold petals and myrrh grains, is doubly effective.

Ingredients
30ml/2 tbsp dried marigold petals
small tin of simple, preferably unperfumed talcum powder
30ml/2 tbsp fine grains or powdered myrrh

1 Grind the marigold petals to a powder, using a pestle and mortar or electric grinder, and mix them into the talcum powder with the myrrh.

2 Return the new mixture to the talcum powder tin, or it may be easier to keep it in a wide-necked jar or pot with a lid. Keep the lid closed to stop contamination of the contents.

3 After drying the feet carefully, use cotton wool balls to dust the feet with the powder, paying special attention to the areas between the toes.

Boils and Abscesses

A boil, also known as a skin abscess, is a localized infection under the skin, which forms a tender, hard swelling. As the body fights the infection, the swelling softens and fills with pus, which is then expelled, sometimes spontaneously and sometimes by lancing. Most small, simple boils can be treated at home, but any that become painful, or do not respond rapidly, should be referred to a doctor. You should also seek medical attention if you are taking any other medication, if there is any fever, or if the boils are associated with diabetes or a damaged immune system illness.

Causes of boils

Boils frequently occur as a result of being run down, either by stress or through poor diet and hygiene. Specific causes include:
• An ingrown hair.
• A splinter or other foreign body in the skin.
• Plugged sweat glands that become infected (acne boils).
• A break in the skin, such as a cut or graze, which becomes infected.
• Depressed immune system, diabetes or other serious illness.

Generally, treatments are geared initially to bringing the boil to a head and allowing it to burst and discharge the pus. It is important that all external applications are as clean as possible – for example, use sterile dressings for applying any poultices. In the medium to longer term, the natural therapies are ideally suited to cleaning the system as a whole, building up immunity to further outbreaks and restoring health and vitality.

Internal treatments

These are aimed at strengthening the immune system.
• **Garlic** may be helpful, for its antibiotic properties and as an immune system booster. Take it regularly in food or as capsules. (Do not take in medicinal doses without professional healthcare advice if on blood-thinning or other medication.)

• Burdock (*Arctium lappa*) and **dandelion root** (*Taraxacum officinale*), taken together as a decoction, have blood-cleansing properties.
• **Cleavers** (*Galium aparine*) or **red clover** (*Trifolium pratense*) can be taken as teas.

Poultices

Many herbs are soothing and anti-inflammatory when used as a hot poultice; two excellent herbs to use in this way are slippery elm (*Ulmus rubra*) and marshmallow (*Althaea officinalis*).
• Marshmallow poultice is made by either pouring boiling water on to some fresh leaves or mixing the powdered root with hot water to make a paste. It may be helpful to use a little oil on the skin first to stop the poultice sticking. The herb should then be placed on the boil or abscess and covered with a clean gauze or strips of cotton, to hold it in position. It can be kept in place until cool, then replaced.
• Slippery elm (*Ulmus rubra*) has been called the "herbalist's knife" for its ability to bring a boil to bursting point. Simply thicken the

Below *The healing powers of slippery elm powder are combined with the antiseptic properties of thyme to make this poultice.*

powder with a little boiling water and apply the paste, as hot as you can bear. Alternatively, combine slippery elm and thyme as in the recipe below: thyme is a good herb to use for its antiseptic, antibacterial properties.

SLIPPERY ELM AND THYME POULTICE

Lay this soothing poultice on the boil while it is still warm, applying a little base oil to the skin first. When the boil has burst, wash the area with a cooled lavender infusion.

Ingredients

small handful of thyme (*Thymus vulgaris*)
boiling water
30ml/2 tbsp slippery elm powder (*Ulmus rubra*)

1 Strip the thyme leaves from the stalks (there should be about 15g/½oz), put them on a saucer and cover with boiling water. Mash thoroughly and leave to cool.

2 Pour off some of the liquid, then add the slippery elm powder and mix thoroughly to make a coarse-textured paste.

3 Apply directly to the skin or enclose in gauze, and hold in place with a bandage.

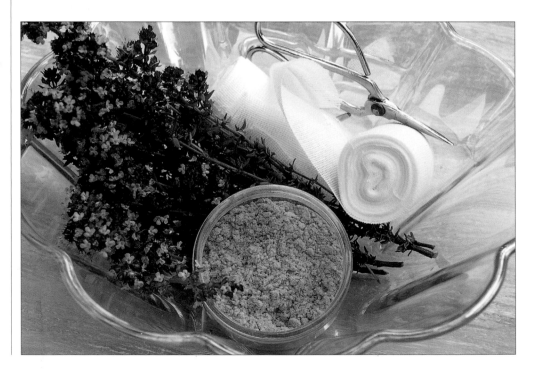

Cold Sores

These are caused by the *Herpes simplex* virus and occur on the lip or just above or below it. They can only be caught through close contact with someone else who has the condition. It is thought that most people carry the virus responsible for cold sores, which is acquired in childhood then lies dormant indefinitely until triggered, though many never have more than one attack. When activated, it causes a tingling sensation on the lip before the itchy, painful sore erupts.

Attack triggers

The virus inhabits the nerves supplying the skin, awaiting an opportunity to become active when the body's defences are lowered or compromised. Common triggers include the following:
- The common cold, flu and other respiratory infections.
- Being generally run down or over-tired.
- Stress and emotional upsets.
- Extremes of temperature.
- Overexposure to cold wind.
- Overexposure to bright sunlight.

When an attack does occur, one or more small blisters erupt on the lips or at the corners of the mouth. These form a crust

Below A healthy diet, rich in vitamins and minerals, strengthens the immune system and makes the eruption of cold sores and other problems less likely.

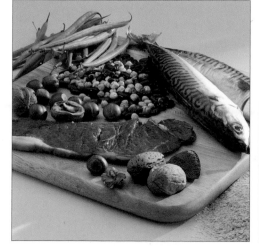

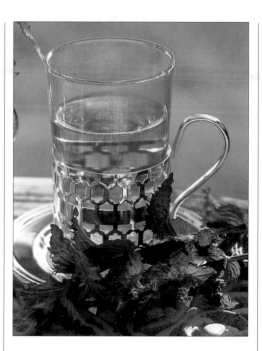

*Above A tea made with freshly picked lemon balm (*Melissa officinalis*) leaves is helpful for relieving the discomfort of cold sores.*

and remain moist underneath for up to 10 days or so before drying out. They are highly contagious during the moist and weeping stages, and contact with others, especially young children, should be avoided.

Avoid known triggers and keep the immune system strong by eating a healthy diet, rich in vitamins A, C and E, zinc and iron.

Below Tinctures can be applied to the affected area on cotton wool (cotton balls) or as cold compresses.

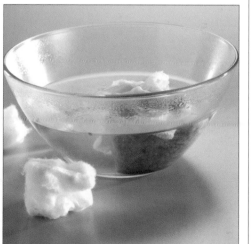

- **Garlic** (*Allium sativum*) also strengthens the immune system, and can be included in food or taken as capsules.
- **Lemon balm** (*Melissa officinalis*) has antiviral properties and is a first-choice herb for dealing with cold sores. Take it as a tea made with the fresh herb, or make a strong infusion and use it to bathe the affected area. (Always wash your hands after touching a cold sore).

Tinctures

Local applications of herbs are most effective when applied in tincture form, dabbed on to the cold sores frequently to dry and heal the area. Lavender, marigold and myrrh are all good for this purpose. You can also use distilled witch hazel.

Compress

A cold compress helps relieve any pain and encourages healing of the skin. Use any of the above tinctures, or distilled witch hazel, diluted in a little water.

You could also make a compress with a strong infusion of rosemary, thyme and peppermint: use 5ml/1tsp of each herb and infuse in 300ml/½ pint/1 cup boiling water for 10 minutes, then strain the liquid off the herbs and cool before applying to the cold sore.

Below Healing lavender oil tincture is simple to prepare at home. It can be dabbed directly on to a cold sore or applied in a compress.

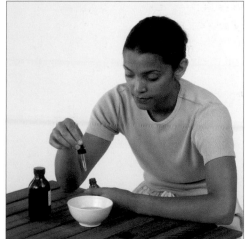

Eye Strain

Tired eyes are a common problem for those who have to spend long hours in front of computer screens or who work in air-conditioned offices under artificial light. Prolonged spells of close work, including reading and writing, can also strain the eyes, and there are a number of simple herbal treatments that will revive and revitalize them. All these treatments involve lying down with your eyes covered for at least 15 minutes, and this enforced relaxation is probably almost as important a part of the treatment as the compresses.

Compresses

Placing a cool herbal compress over the eyes will refresh them, reduce puffiness and relieve itchiness. Keep decoctions or infusions in the refrigerator for an hour before use, to make sure they are cold. Lie down for 15–20 minutes with the pads over the eyes.
• **Fennel** (*Foeniculum vulgare*) – Make a decoction of fennel seeds by boiling 10ml/ 2 tsp seeds in 300ml/½ pint/1¼ cups purified water in a covered pan for 20 minutes. Strain and leave to cool, then use to soak cotton wool pads.
• **Chamomile** (*Chamomaelum nobile*) – Use chamomile teabags to make an infusion, or

Below *Potatoes, cucumber and herbal teabags make useful eye pads.*

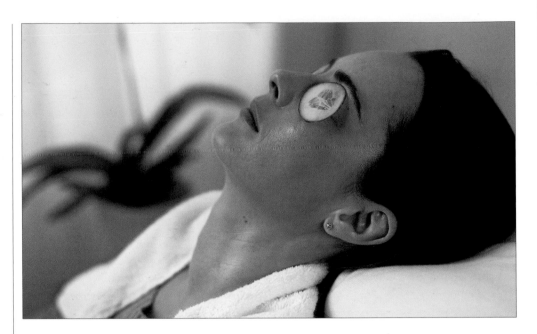

the fresh flowers. In either case, leave to steep for 20 minutes before straining off the liquid and discarding the flowers.
• **Rosewater**: Soak cotton wool pads in an infusion of scented rose petals made with purified water.
• Tea contains tannin, which is astringent and will firm the skin. Place two teabags on a saucer and pour hot water over them. Leave to cool, then refrigerate until cold. Squeeze the excess moisture from the teabags and lie down with them covering your eyes for 10–15 minutes. Remove and gently pat the skin dry before dabbing on moisturizer.

Below *Everyday teabags make good compresses for sore eyes.*

Above *This is the simplest treatment of all. Place a slice of cucumber over each eye while you relax for 15 minutes. The cucumber will very gently tone the skin around the eyes and help restore tired eyes. A rest from close work always helps.*

Below *An old country remedy for tired skin around the eyes is to grate potato finely and place it between two layers of muslin (cheesecloth) before applying it as a compress over the eyes. Certainly, the starch in the potatoes seems to tighten the skin, so it may be more than an old wives' tale.*

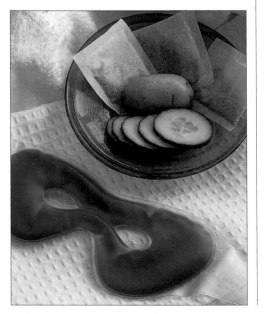

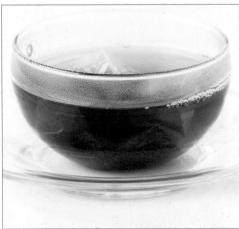

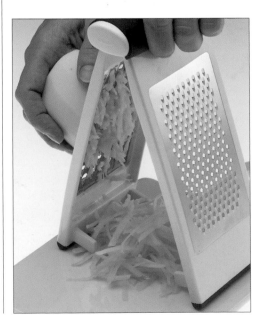

Styes

A stye develops when the root of an eyelash becomes infected. It starts as a tender, red area and then forms a small painful abscess. Repeated attacks may occur If the infection is spread from one lash to another, or if the immune system is depressed, increasing vulnerability to infection. Recurrent styes are occasionally a symptom of diabetes. Always seek medical attention if they are very painful or recur frequently.

Preventive measures
• Eat a healthy diet rich in vitamins and minerals.
• Make sure you get plenty of restful sleep.
• Try to reduce stress.
• Do not share towels, eye make-up or applicators, as styes are contagious.
• Pay scrupulous attention to hygiene.
• Try not to rub the eyes as this will spread the infection.

Herbal tea
• Red clover (*Trifolium pratense*) and fresh red rose petals is a combination that makes a pleasant-tasting, detoxifying drink. Red clover is recommended to boost the body's immune system, helping to defend against infections such as styes.

   Put 20g/⅔oz fresh or 10g/⅓oz dried red clover flowers and 10g/⅓oz fresh red rose petals into a pot. Pour over 600ml/1 pint/ 2½ cups boiling water and leave to infuse for 5 minutes; strain before drinking.

Below *Rose petals are gently soothing.*

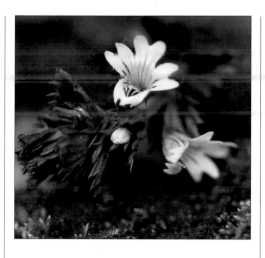

Above *Eyebright (*Euphrasia officinalis*) is a herb traditionally used in eye washes and treatments for styes and conjunctivitis.*

Compress
Applying a warm compress – a piece of gauze dipped in a hot herbal infusion of eyebright (*Euphrasia officinalis*), chamomile (*Matricaria recutita*) or elderflower (*Sambucus nigra*) – helps reduce discomfort, and should bring the stye to a head, releasing the pus.

   To make a soothing rose and elderflower compress, mix 5ml/1 tsp tincture of elderflower with 150ml/6fl oz distilled rosewater and 150ml/6fl oz purified water, warm it gently and apply to the eyelid on gauze or a cotton wool pad.

Below *Getting enough sleep has many health benefits and is essential if you are feeling run down due to a depressed immune system.*

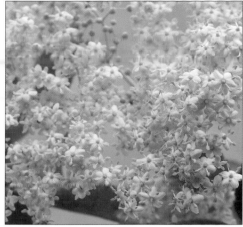

Above *Elderflower (*Sambucus nigra*) has a gentle action when used in a warm compress to reduce the discomfort of a stye.*

Tincture
Echinacea tincture, bought as a ready-made product and taken for a week or two only, may help to give the immune system a general boost.

Steam inhalation
Fill a basin with boiling water, add 2 drops tea tree essential oil, close the eyes and lean over the steam for a minute or two with the head and the basin covered by a towel. Repeat for 5–10 minutes in total at any one time and then on a daily basis until the problem clears.

Below *Tea tree oil is a powerful antiseptic. Add it to a bowl of steaming water as a treatment for styes.*

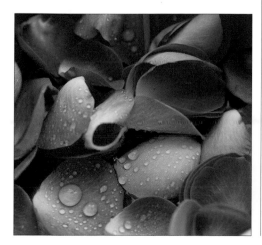

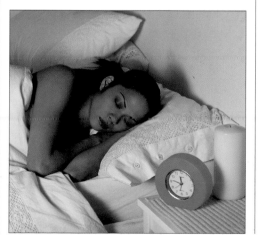

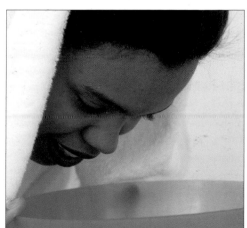

Menopausal Problems

The change of life, when periods cease, is a variable experience. For some women there is very little disturbance to their lives, except for the relief of no longer having monthly bleeding, although the majority probably suffer at least some degree of discomfort. For others, symptoms such as hot flushes, anxiety, depression, insomnia, heavy periods or severe vaginal dryness make their lives miserable for a considerable time. Everyone is different. Don't hesitate to get advice suited to your individual needs.

Hormone replacement therapy

The risks and benefits of taking HRT as a conventional treatment are constantly under review, and different recommendations emerge as new studies are carried out. Clearly there are pros and cons, and it does not suit everyone, so it is worth looking at other ways of helping the process.

Herbs that help

Many herbs have quite powerful hormonal effects (the contraceptive pill itself was originally derived from a species of Mexican yam) and it is always best to seek professional healthcare advice before deciding which ones to take.

All the herbs mentioned here are effective because they are potent, so treat them with respect and follow the safety guidelines given in this book. Do not exceed recommended doses, and if in doubt speak to your doctor before taking them.
• **Sage** (*Salvia officinalis*) is not only a tonic for the nervous system but also has oestrogenic activity and can ease the dramatic drop in hormone levels that can upset the whole system. It helps to reduce excessive sweating.

Make it as a standard tea and drink two small cups daily for 3 weeks, then avoid for at least a week. It is pleasanter sweetened with a teaspoon of honey and will help to reduce night sweats if taken just before going to bed.

Purple sage can be used as well as the common form, but avoid other ornamental varieties of sage.

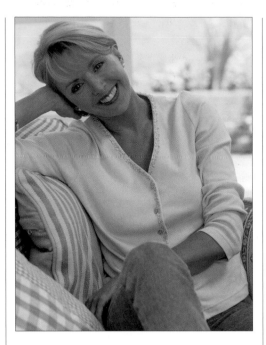

CAUTION Sage can be toxic at high doses or if taken over long periods. It should be avoided if pregnancy is a possibility.

• **Motherwort** (*Leonurus cardiaca*) is a stately plant with delicate mauve flowers. It has a calming action, improving and toning the circulation and helping to relieve

Below *Motherwort has a calming action.*

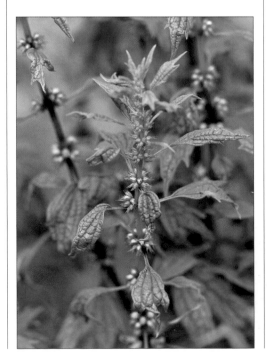

CAUTION Chaste tree may interfere with other medication, including HRT. Too high a dose can induce an itching sensation on the skin. Always seek professional advice immediately if you suffer any adverse reaction, are on other medication or if in any doubt as to the suitability of this herb for your needs.

Left *Herbal remedies offer a way to reduce menopausal discomfort.*

menstrual and menopausal symptoms. It may help to reduce blood pressure, and following one set of clinical trials was said to strengthen the heart. Motherwort can be made into a syrup: take 5ml/1 tsp daily for a week or two, or use it to sweeten sage tea.
• **Chaste tree** (*Vitex agnus-castus*) is another powerful herb with hormonal effects, which may help to relieve symptoms such as hot flushes and night sweats.

CAUTION In high doses motherwort can be a uterine stimulant and should be avoided if pregnancy is a possibility.

Below *Sage is oestrogenic in action.*

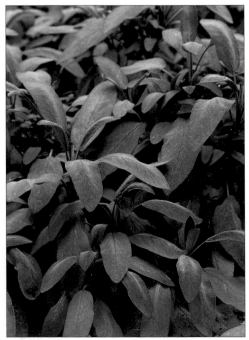

The berry is the part used and it acts on the pituitary gland. Chaste tree is best taken as a ready-made tincture or tablet, when periods first become irregular. Follow the manufacturer's directions or consult a qualified herbalist for advice on dosage to suit your individual requirements.

Herbal teas

Simple relaxants such as chamomile (*Matricaria recutita* and *Chamaemelum nobile*) and lime blossom (*Tilia europaea*), taken as teas 2–3 times a day, may help to reduce the emotional swings that sometimes occur during the menopause.

• For alleviating night sweats try sage (*Salvia officinalis*) and motherwort (*Leonurus cardiaca*) tea. Put 5ml/1 tsp each of dried motherwort and dried sage in a pot and pour on 600ml/1 pint/2½ cups boiling water. Leave to steep for 5–6 minutes then strain and sweeten with honey.

Essential oils

Geranium and rose essential oils seem to have a regulating, balancing effect on the female hormone cycle. Bergamot, neroli and jasmine are all uplifting aromas and can help a great deal with the emotional swings and

Below *Switch to drinking herbal teas. Chamomile and lime blossom are relaxing and help regulate mood swings.*

Right *Rose otto, peppermint and cypress oils are useful for hot flushes. Make up a mix and use it in an atomizer during the day whenever you need to cool down.*

other life changes that may occur around the time of menopause, which can result in a general sense of upheaval and loss.

All these oils can be used either by adding a few drops to the bath or by diluting them in a base oil and massaging into the skin. They can also be vaporized in an essential oil burner.

Try ringing the changes and do not use one oil exclusively for more than a week or so. If you are drawn to the scent of a particular essential oil, then it is most likely to be what you need at that time.

Aromatherapists also recommend the use of clary sage to alleviate hot flushes and night sweats.

Rose otto spray

A cooling spray is handy to counteract the discomfort of hot flushes, which can strike at any time. Rose otto is considered the queen of all essential oils. It has a gentle action and also helps with loss of libido. Put 8–10 drops rose otto

Below *Roses have a gentle action on the skin and a soothing fragrance that can lift the spirits at a difficult time.*

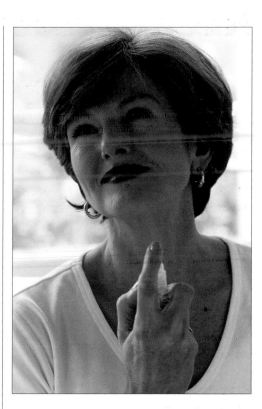

essential oil and 300ml/½ pint/1¼ cups spring water in a screw top bottle. Fit the lid, shake well and transfer some to a small purse-size atomizer that you can carry with you. For a more invigorating mix, use 5 drops peppermint and 3 drops cypress oil.

Below *The exquisite scent of jasmine is uplifting and balancing. Use the essential oil to boost your confidence.*

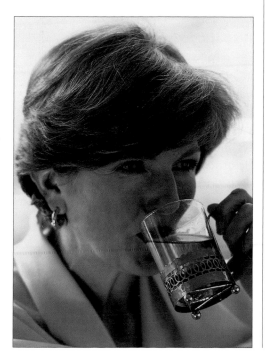

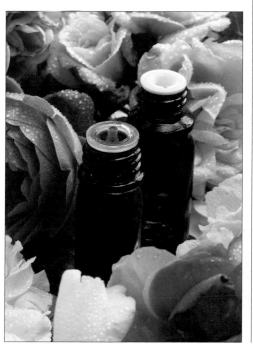

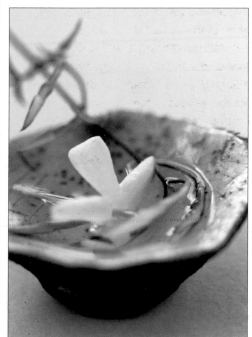

Burns

Herbal first aid is appropriate for minor burns and scalds only, when it can be used to minimize pain and encourage healing. The immediate treatment, before using any herbal preparations, should be to apply cold water for 5–10 minutes, to reduce the heat in the affected tissue. Severe burns require urgent medical assistance, with no delay in getting treatment, especially for children or babies. If the burn is from a chemical, affected clothing can be removed, but if clothing is stuck to the burn, it is better not to remove it before seeking treatment as this might do more damage.

> **CAUTION** Burns larger than the palm of your hand should be seen by a doctor immediately, regardless of any self-help treatment that has been advised here. All burns are painful and should be touched as little as possible.

Tips for treating burns

Remember, do not use greasy ointments, butter or other fats on new burns as all this does is fry the skin. Always cool the area thoroughly as the first treatment.

Below *Lavender essential oil, applied directly to the affected skin, has been found to be very effective in healing burns.*

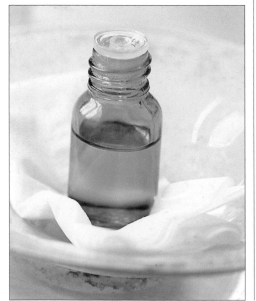

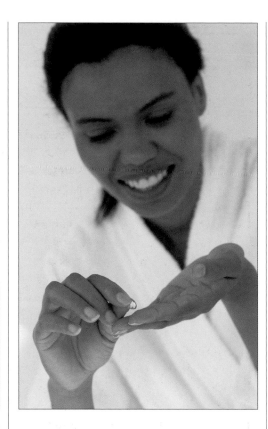

Above *Vitamin E oil, squeezed from a capsule and applied to a burn, supports the skin and reduces scarring.*

Once the skin has been cooled a valuable home remedy is honey: this is both antiseptic and promotes healing. Once healing has started, a vitamin E cream can aid restoration of tissue elasticity and

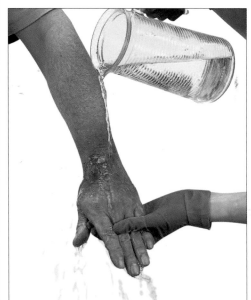

reduce scarring. Do not give hot drinks to someone who has a burn; frequent small sips of cool water can help to replace lost fluids in more serious cases.

Essential oils

Lavender essential oil has anti-inflammatory, analgesic properties and promotes healing of the tissues. It has been used as an effective first-aid treatment for burns since the early years of the 20th century, when René Gattefossé, the founding father of aromatherapy, fortuitously discovered its miraculous healing powers following a laboratory accident.

Provided – and this is crucial – you use a top quality, unadulterated, pure lavender essential oil, a few drops can be applied directly to the skin. If a larger area is affected, the oil can be put on to sterile gauze or smooth lint first.

Tea tree oil may help to prevent blistering of the skin: dilute 1–2 drops of the oil in 5ml/1tsp water and apply it to a minor burn, after first cooling it with plain water.

Other herbal treatments

An aloe vera plant is an invaluable source of first aid for minor burns and scalds. (The plant is easy to care for provided it is kept frost-free and given a sunny spot, such as a kitchen windowsill.) Simply break open one of the leaves and spread the thick gel that seeps out directly on to the burn. If this is done as soon as possible it will promote scar-free healing. Alternatively, an infusion of chamomile (*Matricaria recutita* or *Chamaemelum nobile*) or pot marigold (*Calendula officinalis*) can be applied to a burn on a smooth dressing.

Marigold skin salve (see Skin Irritations) may be used after some time has elapsed and the skin is beginning to heal, to ease continuing inflammation and soreness.

Left *Pouring cold water over a burn to reduce the heat is the first step to take when applying first aid. If the burn is in a suitable area such as a hand or arm it can be held under cold running water.*

Sunburn

Sunlight produces a sense of well-being and we all need a little exposure to sun in order to metabolize vitamin D. Too much, however, is not only ageing, but increases the possibility of developing skin cancer. Prevention is always better than cure, and strong sunshine should be avoided at all costs. Some people burn more easily than others (those with fair skins are particularly at risk) and if mild sunburn does occur, herbal preparations can be used to soothe the discomfort and aid the skin to heal and recover.

The risk of skin cancer

An increasingly frequent sequel to excessive exposure to the sun is skin cancer, and the reductions in the earth's ozone layer make this likely to become dramatically more common in future years, even in countries some distance away from the Equator.

The sun has an ageing effect on the skin, so enjoy it but use good suntan and aftersun moisturizing creams and keep out of the midday sun. Sunbeds can damage skin. They do not protect against sunburn; you still need to be careful when out in hot sunshine.

Below Take sensible precautions to minimize exposure to sunlight, such as covering up when you are out and about and staying out of the sun during the hottest part of the day.

Compress

For a mild case of sunburn, start by cooling areas of red skin, as for minor burns. Applying a chilled infusion of chamomile (*Chamaemelum nobile*), elderflower (*Sambucus nigra*) or lavender (*Lavandula* spp) flowers, as a compress, is very soothing. Cooled distilled witch hazel (*Hamamelis virginiana*) also makes a good compress.

Poultice

Strawberries and yogurt both take the heat out of sunburnt skin. Mash them up together (make sure you use plain yogurt) and apply directly to the skin as a poultice, keeping it in place with a piece of gauze or cotton fabric.

Essential oils

Lavender essential oil may be used as for burns, directly on the skin; if you are not sure of its purity, dilute it (adding 5 drops to a small bowl of water) and carefully dab it on to the skin. Chamomile essential oil, also diluted, may be similarly used, but only on unbroken skin.

Either of these oils could also be added to the bath (5–8 drops); make sure the water is

Below right Rose and chamomile are good essential oils to use on sun-damaged skin. Put a few drops in bath water.

no more than tepid, as a hot bath would make the problem worse.

Marigold skin salve (see Skin Irritations) is a useful all-purpose cream to apply to sun-reddened skin, after first cooling it with a herbal infusion.

Routine after-sun care

Essential oils of rose, chamomile, lavender or sandalwood make excellent aftercare for leathery, sun-damaged skin. Dilute any one of these in a base oil, such as sweet almond, (adding 2–3 drops to 5ml/1 tsp base oil) and massage in gently twice a day. Rose oil, although it is expensive, is probably the best one to choose: it is safe to use on sensitive skins, provided it is a pure essential oil and not synthetic.

After-sun treatment

• For a refreshing spray to use after exposure to the sun, mix 8 drops rose oil in 25ml/5 tsp water and apply with an atomizer.
• For a soothing and cooling oil for sunburnt skin mix 5 drops each of rose essential oil and chamomile essential oil together with 45ml/3 tbsp each grapeseed oil and virgin olive oil and 15ml/1 tbsp wheatgerm oil. Combine all the oils in a bowl. Massage gently into the sun-reddened area.

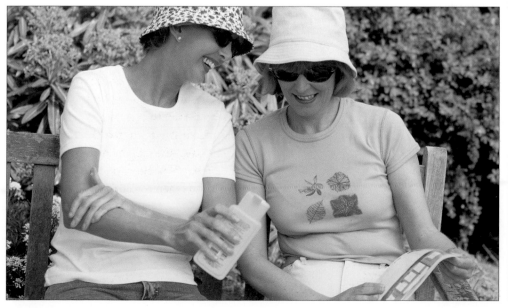

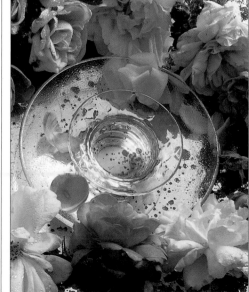

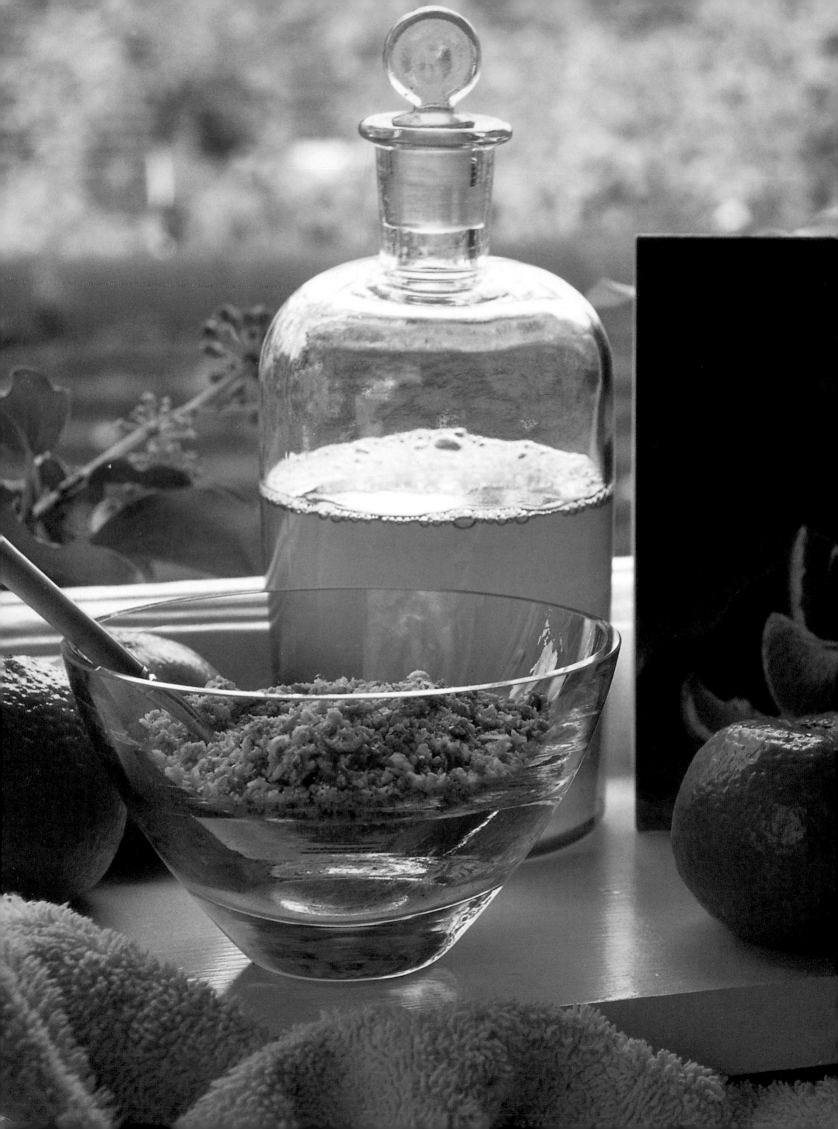

Herbal Beauty Treatments

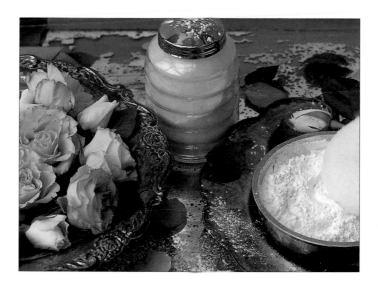

Using simple beauty treatments made with herbs, flowers and basic natural ingredients contributes greatly to general health and well-being. Many commercial beauty products contain parabens and other chemicals, which studies have found could have an injurious effect on the system, so it makes sense to find alternatives where practicable. The recipes in this chapter show how to make your own hair products and face creams, body lotions, dusting powders and many other items for daily hygiene and general beauty care. They are easy to follow and the products take little time to prepare. It is important to follow guidelines on how to store them and how long they should be kept.

Above *Fragrant dusting powder scented with herbal flowers is a luxurious beauty treat with which to pamper yourself.*

Left *Beauty preparations can be made with a variety of natural ingredients.*

Healthy Hair

Modern hair care products can make your hair look good, but many of them contain potentially harmful chemicals that you may prefer to avoid. Using the same ones consistently can also lead to build-up on hair and scalp, so it makes sense to give your hair a rest by using herbal treatments and natural ingredients, which have been tried and tested and provide a simpler way to keep hair in top condition.

Herbal shampoo

This is the most difficult hair-care item to produce in "natural" form. All commercial shampoos contain some form of detergent, which may strip the hair of its natural oils, but also have an effective cleansing action.

The easiest way to make a "herbal" shampoo that will leave your hair clean and shiny is to add 2–3 drops essential oil to 15ml/1 tbsp ready-made organic shampoo base (available from specialist suppliers); or you could mix the shampoo base with an equal quantity of a strong herbal infusion. A mild, fragrance-free, pH-balanced shampoo can be used as a base.

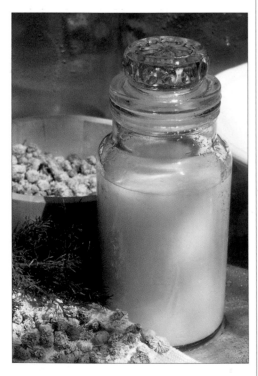

Above *Herbal shampoo has a gentle, less abrasive action than commercial shampoo.*

HAIR RESCUER

This rich, nourishing formula helps to improve the condition of dry and damaged hair.

Ingredients

Makes enough for 1 treatment
30ml/2 tbsp olive oil
30ml/2 tbsp light sesame oil
2 eggs
30ml/2 tbsp coconut milk
30ml/2 tbsp runny honey
5ml/1 tsp coconut oil

1 Combine all the ingredients together in a blender or food processor, until smooth.

2 Transfer to a bottle. Keep refrigerated and use within 3 days.

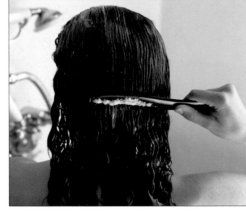

3 Comb the mixture through your hair after shampooing, leave for 5 minutes.

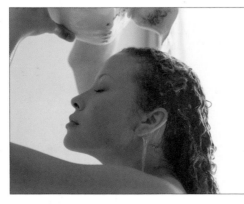

4 Rinse the hair with warm water and gently rub dry with a towel.

Conditioners and herbal rinses

The best way to keep hair looking glossy is to use a natural conditioner followed by a herbal rinse. Oil-based preparations need to be used before shampooing; lighter ones made of natural ingredients can be used after a shampoo and washed out with warm water and a herbal rinse. For dry to normal hair try a mixture of avocado and egg, for oily hair yogurt makes a good conditioner.

To revive dry or sun-damaged hair, an oil-based treatment, rich in essential oils, works best.

NETTLE RINSE FOR DANDRUFF

This herbal rinse helps to keep the hair shiny and in good condition. Make it freshly the evening before you wash your hair.

Ingredients

25g/1oz fresh nettle leaves (*Urtica dioica*)
25g/1oz nasturtium flowers and leaves
1 litre/1¾ pints/4 cups water
30ml/2 tbsp cider vinegar
30ml/2 tbsp distilled witch hazel

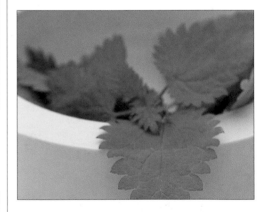

1 Put the nettles and nasturtium flowers and leaves in a heatproof bowl. Boil the water and pour it over the nettles and nasturtiums. (Nettles lose their sting in boiling water.)

2 Leave to stand overnight. Strain off the herbs and add the vinegar and witch hazel.

3 Hold your head over a portable bowl as you pour the rinse through your hair. Keep pouring the rinse from the bowl back into the pitcher and re-apply at six times.

CHAMOMILE RINSE FOR FAIR HAIR

Combined with cider vinegar, chamomile and rosemary have been used in hair rinses for hundreds of years. The herbs enhance hair colour and the vinegar is a wonderful scalp conditioner. Chamomile has long been favoured by blondes for their fair hair; although it does not bleach, it enhances the hair's natural colour.

Ingredients

Makes enough for 3 treatments
50g/2oz dried chamomile (*Chamaemelum nobile*) flowers
900ml/1½ pints boiling water
50ml/2fl oz cider vinegar
5 drops chamomile essential oil

1 Put the chamomile flowers into a wide-necked jar and pour the water on top.

2 Seal the jar and leave to stand overnight. Strain the infusion repeatedly through muslin (cheesecloth) or paper coffee filters, until it is clear.

3 Add the cider vinegar and essential oil. Store in a stoppered glass bottle in the refrigerator and use within a week, as a final rinse when washing your hair.

ROSEMARY RINSE FOR DARK HAIR

Fresh rosemary has a high essential oil content and is also beneficial for dry hair.

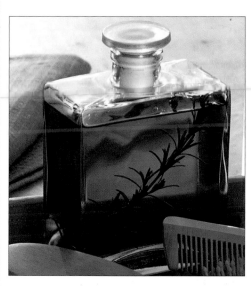

Ingredients

40g/1½oz fresh rosemary (*Rosmarinus officinalis*)
1 litre/1¾ pints/4 cups boiling water
50ml/2fl oz cider vinegar

Make as for the chamomile rinse.
Use frequently for shiny hair.

Below *Herbal rinses add gloss and shine.*

WARM OIL HAIR TREATMENT

Use this treatment once a month to improve the hair texture and to condition the scalp.

Ingredients

Makes enough for 5 treatments
90ml/6 tbsp coconut oil
3 drops rosemary essential oil
2 drops tea tree essential oil
2 drops lavender essential oil

1 Gently warm the coconut oil in a bowl over hot water until it melts, then mix in the rest of the ingredients.

2 Apply sparingly, while still warm, to dry hair; the head should not be saturated. Massage it in before covering your head with a hot towel for 20 minutes.

3 Shampoo as normal. Reheat the remaining oil for subsequent uses.

Below *The regular use of herbal conditioners gives hair a healthy gleam.*

Below far left *A chamomile rinse adds a sheen to fair hair. Herbal hair care is gentler on the scalp and will not cause the chemical build-up associated with commercial products.*

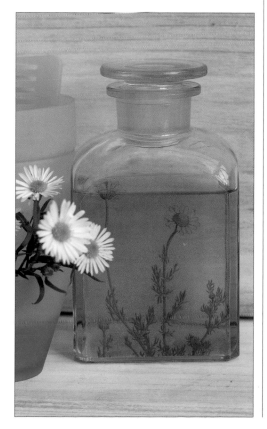

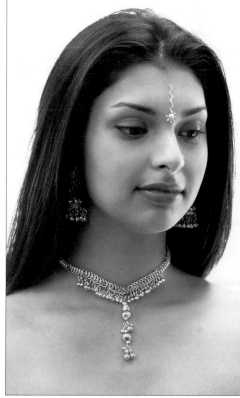

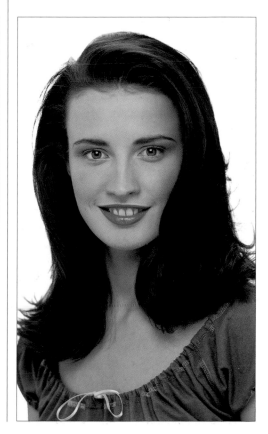

Eyes and Lips

The skin around the eyes is the most delicate on the face and the first to show signs of tiredness or stress. Eye creams can make matters worse, especially if their texture is too heavy; there is also a tendency to drag the skin when applying them. Simple herbal compresses are the best way to revive and revitalize tired eyes, and the relaxation involved in lying down with the eyes closed and gently covered is a bonus.

CHAMOMILE COMPRESS

This is a tried and tested treatment for tired eyes. Although it can be done using herbal teabags, if you have time it is worth making the compresses from muslin (cheesecloth) and whole chamomile flowers rather than the more powdery mix that often goes into teabags. Whether you are using cloth bags or teabags, cover them with boiling water, leave them to cool, then put them in the refrigerator to get cold. Lie down for 20 minutes with the compresses over the eyes.

Ingredients

5g/⅕ oz chamomile (*Chamaemelum nobile*) flowers
2 x 15cm/6in square unbleached muslin
20cm/8in fine ribbon or string.

Place a handful of chamomile flowers in the centre of each muslin square. Gather the muslin into a bundle and tie it with ribbon or string.

Below *A compress made with chamomile flowers is restful for tired eyes.*

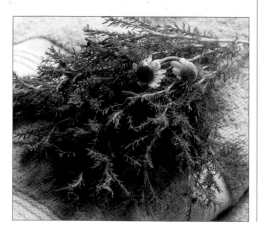

LAVENDER LIP BALM

It is quite simple to make your own soothing cream for lips chapped by weather or illness. Beeswax and cocoa butter are rich emollients; wheatgerm oil, with its high vitamin E content, is a powerful antioxidant and lavender essential oil is well known for its healing ability. You can also apply a simple mixture of honey and rosewater as a salve for sore or chapped lips.

Ingredients

5ml/1 tsp beeswax
5ml/1 tsp cocoa butter
5ml/1 tsp wheatgerm oil
5ml/1 tsp almond oil
3 drops lavender essential oil

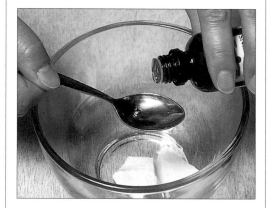

1 Put the beeswax into a small bowl and add the cocoa butter, wheatgerm oil and almond oil. Set the bowl over a pan of simmering water.

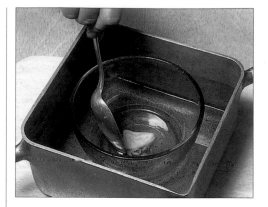

2 Stir the mixture constantly until the beeswax has melted.

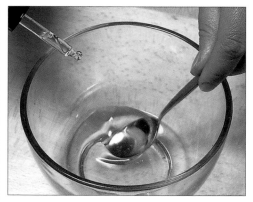

3 Remove the bowl from the heat and allow the mixture to cool for a few minutes before mixing in the lavender oil. Pour into a small jar and leave to set.

Below *Lavender lip balm is rich and soothing with a pleasant scent.*

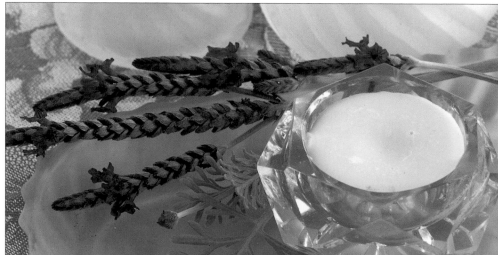

Teeth and Fresh Breath

Herbs can be used in many ways to keep the breath fresh and the teeth clean. Although you may not wish to use a herbal tooth powder all the time, it does provide a viable, natural alternative to manufactured products, which may contain a long list of synthetic chemical ingredients.

Simple teeth cleansers

• **Sage** (*Salvia officinalis*) – Rub teeth with fresh sage leaves.
• **Lemon peel** – Pare the peel off the fruit and rub over the teeth to remove stains.

Simple breath fresheners

• **Parsley, watercress, mint** – Chew the fresh leaves after eating a garlicky meal.
• **Whole spices** – Suck or chew fennel seeds, star anise, angelica, caraway, calamus root, cinnamon stick, or cloves after a meal.
• **Rosewater** – Dilute half-and-half with water for rinsing the mouth.
• **Lavender infusion** – Infuse 15ml/1 tbsp dried lavender (*Lavandula*) in 300ml/½ pint/ 1¼ cups water and use as an oral rinse.

Below Keep the teeth clean and the breath fresh with natural cleansers and rinses.

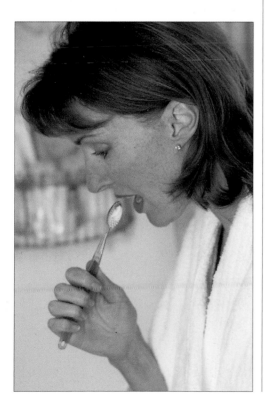

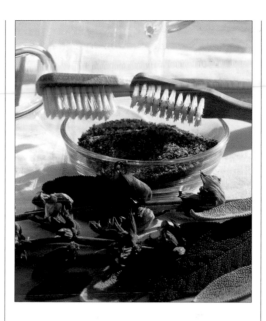

Above Powdered sage and salt make a traditional mixture for cleaning the teeth.

SAGE AND SALT TOOTH POWDER

The cleansing action of sage and salt will make your mouth tingle. Rinse your mouth well with plenty of fresh water after using this tooth powder. For a milder effect, substitute 15ml/1 tbsp orris root powder for the salt.

Ingredients

25g/1oz fresh sage (*Salvia officinalis*) leaves
60ml/4 tbsp sea salt

1 With a pair of scissors, snip the sage leaves into an ovenproof dish.

2 Mix in the salt, grinding it into the leaves with a wooden spoon or pestle. Bake the mixture in a very low oven for about 1 hour, until the sage is dry and crisp.

3 Pound the mixture again until it is reduced to a powder. Keep in a jar in the bathroom and use on a dampened toothbrush instead of toothpaste.

Right Consider incorporating herbal ingredients into a chemical-free range of toiletries. Such products are now more widely available in health food stores and larger supermarkets.

SPICED LEMON VERBENA MOUTHWASH

Commercial antiseptic mouthwashes can upset the natural acid balance of the mouth. A herbal mouthwash is gentler and this one – which is made with tangy lemon verbena – is particularly pleasant to use.

Ingredients

5ml/1 tsp each ground nutmeg (*Myristica fragrans*), ground cloves, cardamom pods and caraway seeds
small handful fresh lemon verbena leaves (*Aloysia triphylla*) or 15g/½ oz dried lemon verbena
600ml/1 pint/2½ cups purified water
30ml/2 tbsp sweet sherry

1 Put the spices and lemon verbena into a pan with the water. Bring to the boil and simmer for 30 minutes.

2 Strain through a sieve (strainer) lined with kitchen paper, then add the sherry and pour into a clean bottle.

3 To use, dilute 15–30ml/1–2 tbsp in a tumbler of water.

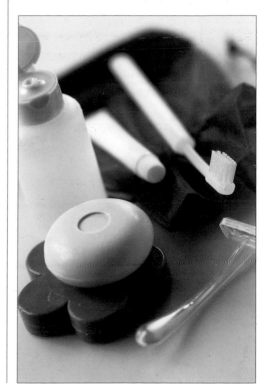

Skin Treatments

The lavish use of a body lotion after a daily bath or shower will help prevent skin drying out and losing its elasticity. Making your own is not difficult and the simple ingredients, flower waters and floral essential oils are nourishing and revitalizing. Both the recipes given here make lotions that will keep for up to 2 months if stored in sealed jars in a cool, dark place.

COCONUT AND ORANGEFLOWER BODY LOTION

This creamy preparation is wonderfully nourishing for dry skin. It is solid at room temperature but melts when lukewarm.

Ingredients
50g/2oz coconut oil
60ml/4 tbsp sunflower oil
10ml/2 tsp wheatgerm oil
10 drops orangeflower essence

1 Put the coconut oil in a bowl over a pan of gently simmering water. Once it has melted, stir in the sunflower and wheatgerm oils.

2 Leave to cool, then add the orangeflower essence and pour into a jar. It will solidify after several hours.

Below *Wheatgerm oil is rich in vitamin E, which protects skin cells against premature aging. Coconut oil is rich and moisturizing.*

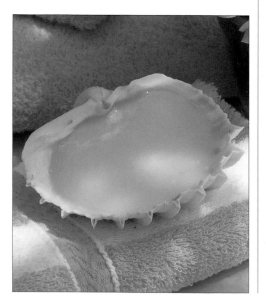

ROSE BODY LOTION

This recipe gives a rich, creamy lotion. If you prefer a runnier, more liquid texture, increase the amount of water in the mixture by 30ml/2 tbsp.

Ingredients
45ml/3 tbsp hot, recently boiled water
2.5ml/½ tsp borax
5ml/1 tsp beeswax
30ml/2 tbsp emulsifying ointment
25ml/5 tsp apricot kernel oil
20ml/4 tsp cold-pressed sunflower oil
10 drops rose essential oil

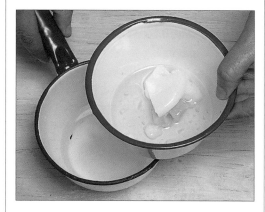

1 Dissolve the borax in the boiled water. Melt the beeswax and emulsifying ointment with the apricot kernel and sunflower oils in a double boiler (or in a bowl set over a pan of simmering water). Remove from the heat once the wax has melted and stir well.

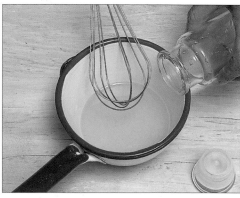

2 Add the borax solution, whisking as you do so. Keep whisking until it cools, then add the rose oil. Pour the lotion into a tinted glass jar, seal and store in a cool place.

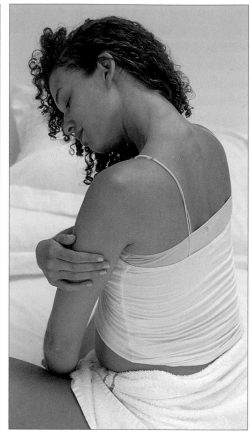

Above *Smoothing on body lotion after a bath or shower moisturizes dry skin and softens rough patches.*

Below *A rose-scented body lotion is ideal for sensitive skins. Make a double quantity, keeping some for yourself to use regularly and some to give away.*

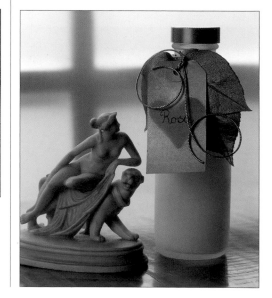

Dusting powder

There is a tendency to think of dusting powders as being the province of bathed babies and elderly ladies, but this needn't be so. A talcum powder, dusted all over the body, is a wonderful way to coat the body with fragrance.

Dusting powders can be made from scratch or you can use unscented talc as a base. Either way you will be able to formulate a scented powder quite different from commercial talcum powders. Dusting powders look wonderful in shallow bowls on a dressing table accompanied by a pretty powder puff.

Single fragrance dusting powders

These dusting powders are the simplest of all to make, especially if your base is ready-made unscented talcum powder. For each 75ml/5 tbsp talc you will need 15ml/1 tbsp cornflour (cornstarch), scented with 5 drops of your favourite essential oil. Fragrance is so personal that you will need to decide for yourself the properties of the different oils, but it is generally accepted that jasmine sets the scene for seduction, roses are romantic and peppermint or lemon are good to use after vigorous exercise at the gym.

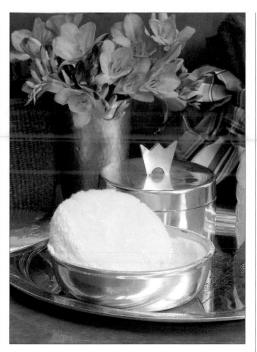

LUSCIOUS LAVENDER BODY POWDER

A soft blend of lavender, coriander and geranium, with a hint of fresh lemon, gives this body powder a delightful fragrance. Use it after your evening bath or shower or when you've been to the gym. The fragrance is better absorbed when the skin is slightly damp and the pores are open. Apply with a powder puff or cotton wool (cotton balls).

Left Fragrant dusting powder makes the skin feel wonderfully soft and smooth.

Ingredients

60ml/4 tbsp white kaolin clay (available from pharmacies) mixed with 60ml/4 tbsp arrowroot and 60ml/4 tbsp cornflour (cornstarch) or 180ml/12tbsp unscented talc
15ml/1 tbsp cornflour
3 drops lavender essential oil
3 drops coriander essential oil
3 drops lemon essential oil
3 drops geranium essential oil

1 Mix together the kaolin clay, arrowroot and cornflour (cornstarch) in a deep bowl, or put the unscented talc in the bowl.

2 Put the 15ml/1 tbsp of cornflour into a separate bowl and add the essential oils. Stir thoroughly.

3 Add the scented cornflour to the larger bowl and mix together thoroughly. Decant into a container.

Below *Lavender body powder has a delicious, light fragrance.*

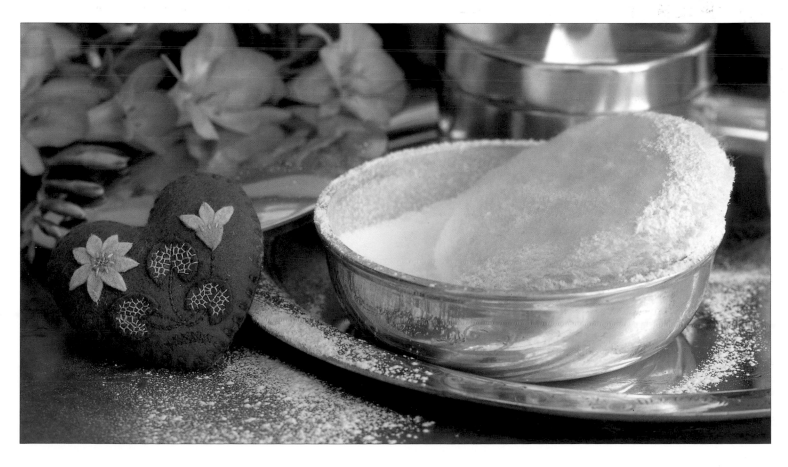

Bathing

Herbal baths provide the ideal way to relax the mind and body, to revive and restore the system. Instead of putting fresh herbs into bath bags, essential oils can be added directly to the water. The occasional use of an exfoliating body scrub will leave skin revitalized and a milk and honey bath oil restores vital nourishment. As a final touch, making your own soap provides the opportunity to incorporate ingredients to suit individual likes and needs.

Below Taking time out to relax in a warm bath is beneficial for mind and body.

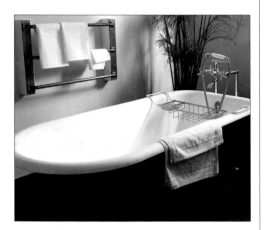

MILK AND HONEY BATH OIL WITH ROSEMARY

Milk is well known for its cleansing and lubricating qualities when applied to the skin. The addition of a little shampoo makes this a dispersing oil, so it does not leave a greasy rim around the bath.

Ingredients
2 eggs
45ml/3 tbsp rosemary herb oil
10ml/2 tsp honey
10ml/2 tsp baby shampoo
15ml/1 tbsp vodka
150ml/¼ pint/⅔ cup milk

1 Beat the eggs and oil together, then add the other ingredients and mix thoroughly. Pour into a clean glass bottle.

2 Add 30–45ml/2–3 tbsp to the bath and keep the rest chilled. Use within 2 days.

Essential oils in the bath

Add 5–6 drops essential oil straight from the bottle directly into a full bath. Do not add while the water is still running as the oil will evaporate too quickly and be wasted. Alternatively, mix two or three essential oils together in a base of sweet almond oil or jojoba oil. Then add 20 drops of the mixed oil to the bath. The quantities given are for a 50ml bottle of base oil.
- **Anti-stress mix**: 10 drops each marjoram, lavender and sandalwood.
- **Invigorating mix**: 5 drops rosemary, 5 drops camphor, 10 drops peppermint.

Stimulating scrubs

Face and body scrubs are increasingly popular as part of a beauty regime. The slightly rough texture of the scrub will efficiently exfoliate and stimulate the skin, leaving it clean and soft and ready for moisturizing. It is also a good idea to exfoliate before applying tanning lotion. Used at any time of the year but especially in the dark, cold months when the body never sees the sun, a scrub will remove dead skin and tone the skin, leaving it looking revitalized, but it should not be used too often, especially on sensitive skins.

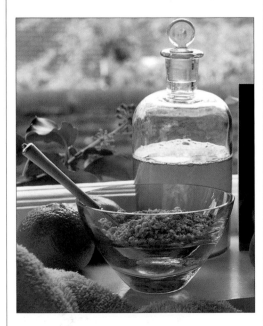

Above *Regular use of a rough-textured body scrub invigorates and smooths the skin.*

CITRUS BODY SCRUB

The slightly gritty texture of this exfoliating scrub provided by ground sunflower seeds, oatmeal, sea salt and orange peel helps to remove dead skin cells and stimulates the blood supply to the skin, leaving you tingling and toned. The combination of the aromatic orange peel and the grapefruit oil gives it a fresh scent.

Ingredients
Makes enough for 5 treatments
45ml/3 tbsp freshly ground sunflower seeds
45ml/3 tbsp medium oatmeal
45ml/3 tbsp flaked sea salt
45ml/3 tbsp finely grated orange peel
3 drops grapefruit essential oil
almond oil, to mix

1 Thoroughly mix all the ingredients except the almond oil and store in a sealed glass jar.

2 Mix to a paste with almond oil before using. Rub over the body, paying particular attention to areas of hard, dry skin such as the elbows, knees and ankles.

3 Remove the residue before showering or bathing.

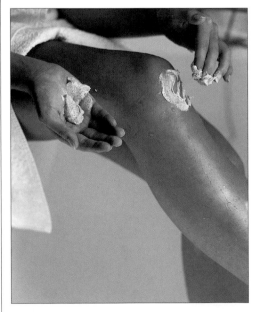

Above *Knees and elbows are prone to dryness so use this body scrub to treat those areas.*

LEMON GRASS SOAP

The toning and antiseptic qualities of lemon grass not only help relieve oily skin and acne, but can also help tighten up post-pregnancy or post-diet skin. Use the soap within a month.

Ingredients

Makes 2 bars

150g/5oz unscented soap (preferably made with vegetable oils)
12 drops lemon grass essential oil

1 Using the finest side of a cheese grater, grate the soap into a bowl.

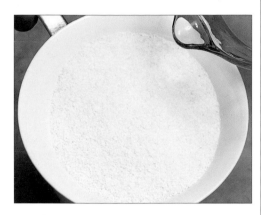

2 Add water to the bowl in the proportion of one part water to two parts soap.

3 Put the bowl over a pan of simmering water and heat the mixture gently, stirring continuously, until it coalesces. You will see this happening slowly and the soap will become thicker, gradually getting harder to stir. Remove the pan from the heat.

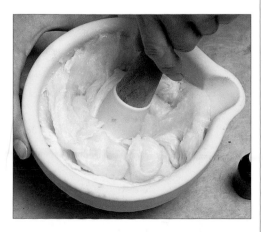

4 Transfer the soap into a pestle and mortar and add the lemon grass oil. Mix well to distribute the oil.

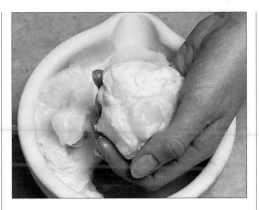

5 With wet hands, take about half the soap and work into a bar.

6 Repeat to make another bar. Leave on a wooden board to dry out and set hard. This may take a couple of days.

Below *For a calming bath, add a handful of neroli-scented calming milk bath mixture and wash with soaps made with pure vegetable oils because they are the kindest to the skin. Lemon grass root is toning and antiseptic in action.*

CALMING MILK BATH MIXTURE

Chamomile and neroli both have many valuable properties, essentially to soothe and calm. Chamomile is a wonderfully gentle herb, used to settle upset stomachs and to treat insomnia; it is also used in beauty preparations to pacify sensitive skin. Neroli oil comes from the flowers of the Seville orange tree and is known to relieve depression, anxiety and insomnia. Add this soothing mixture to a running bath and allow a traditional remedy to soak away the cares of everyday life.

Ingredients

120ml/4fl oz/½ cup fine sea salt
240ml/8fl oz/1 cup powdered milk
6 drops chamomile essential oil
12 drops neroli essential oil

Mix the sea salt, powdered milk and essential oils well. Place in a covered container and leave for 3 weeks for the oils to permeate the ingredients before adding to the bath.

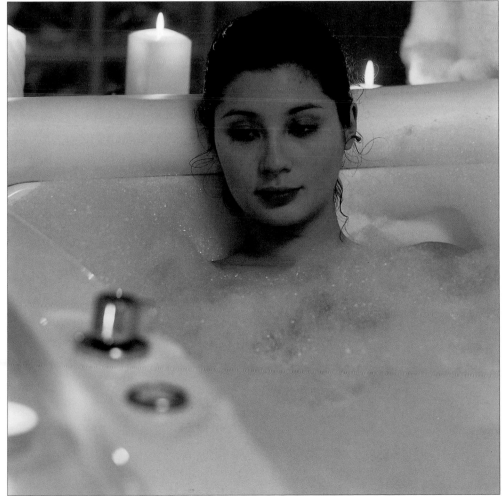

Index

A
abscesses 66
acidity 53
acne 64
aloe vera juice 53
anxiety 38
aromatherapy 24–5
arthritis 74–5
athlete's foot 65

B
bags, revival 42
bath bags 33
    nettle 58
bathing 94–5
beauty treatments 83
bites 76
body lotions 92–3
body scrub, citrus 94
boils 66
breath 89
bruises 78
burns 80

C
calming milk bath mixture
    95
catarrh 50
chaste tree 71, 73
chilblains 60
circulation 58
cleanser, rose 86
cleansing rinse, herbal 64
cocktail for colds and coughs
    48
cold sores 67
colds 46–7, 48
compresses 30
    chamomile 88
    cramp bark and rosemary
        70
    eye pads 51
    herbal eye pads 68
    lavender 44
concentration 41
constipation 56
coughs 48
cramp 61
creams 31
    rose hand cream 90
    tea tree foot cream 91
cuts 77

D
dandruff 85
decoctions 27
    ginger 60
    ginger and lemon 49
depression 40
diarrhoea 57
dosage 10, 13
dusting powders 93

E
eczema 63
energy 42
essential oils 22–3, 24, 25, 32
evening primrose 71
eye strain 68
eyes 88

F
face mask 86
facial care 86–7
feet 91
    cold feet 59
feverfew 45
foot bath
    antifungal 65
    herbal 91
    lemon verbena and lavender 42, 91
    mustard 47
foot powder, marigold and myrrh 65
freezing herbs 19

G
gargle 49
garlic bread 94
genera, plant classification 10–11
ginger, fresh root 54
grazes 77

H
hair 84–5
    hair rescuer 84
hands 90
    cold hands 59
    rose hand mask 90
harvesting herbs 86–7
hayfever 51
headaches 44
health benefits 35
heartburn 53
herbal infusions 26
herbal remedies 6, 9, 37
    safety issues 10–11, 12–13
herbs 14, 15
    dried herbs 20
    growing herbs 16–17
    harvesting and drying 18
    herb salts 19
    herbs in food 34–5
    preserving and storing 19
    wild herbs 14

I
indigestion 52
influenza 46–7

ingredients 20–1
inhalants 32
    essential oil 50
    fresh herb 50

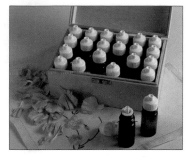

J
juice, ginger with pineapple 52

L
liniment, rheumatism 74
lips 88
    lavender lip balm 88
liquorice 11, 56
lotion
    coconut and orangeflower 92
    rose 92
    sage and myrrh 55

M
massage oils 29, 59
memory 41
menopausal problems 72–3
menstrual problems 70, 71
migraine 45
moisturizer, elderflower 87
morning sickness 54
mouth ulcers 55
mouthwash, spiced lemon verbena 89

N
nails 90
nausea 54

O
oils 21
    after-sun soothing 81
    cold-infused oils 29, 39
    essential oils 22–3, 24, 25, 32
    lavender 39
    milk and honey bath oil with
        rosemary 94
    rose geranium nail oil 90
    sleep time spray 43
    warm infused rosemary oil 59
    warm oil hair treatment 85
ointments 31
    calendula 62
    comfrey bruise ointment 78

P
pharmaceutical drugs 11
poultices 30
    slippery elm and thyme 66

powders 20
    luscious lavender 93
    sage and salt tooth powder 89
pre-menstrual symptoms 71
purées 19

R
rheumatism 74–5
rinse, chamomile 85
    nettle 85
    rosemary 85

S
safety issues 10–11, 12–13
seasonings 34
shampoo 84
skin irritations 62
skin salve, marigold 62
sleep 43
sleep pillows 33
soap, lemongrass 95
sore throats 49
spices 20–1
sprains and strains 79
spray, rose otto 73
spray, sleep time 43
spritzer, kiwi and stem ginger 42
stings 76
stress 39
styes 69
sunburn 81
syrups 27
    garlic cold 46

T
teas
    borage flower 40
    celery seed and parsley 75
    elderflower, yarrow and
        peppermint 50
    fennel seed 53
    ginger 54
    ginger and cinnamon 57
    herb 26, 38
    lemon balm and lime blossom
        39
    lemon verbena 41
    morning after 44
    red clover and rose petal 69
    restorative 40
    sage and motherwort 72
    sleep-inducing 43
    soothing 45
    vervain and lady's mantle 71
teeth 89
tinctures 21, 28
    raspberry leaf 55
tiredness 42
toner, elderflower 86
    rose 86
toning milk, marigold 87

V
vapour rubs 47
vomiting 54

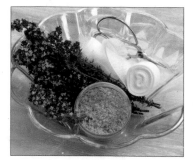